THE INVADING BODY

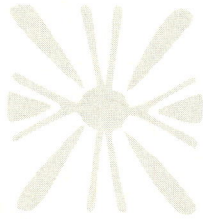

THE INVADING BODY

Reading Illness Autobiographies

EINAT AVRAHAMI

University of Virginia Press
Charlottesville and London

University of Virginia Press
© 2007 by the Rector and Visitors of the University of Virginia
All rights reserved
Printed in the United States of America on acid-free paper
First published 2007

1 3 5 7 9 8 6 4 2

LIBRARY OF CONGRESS CATALOGING-IN-PUBLICATION DATA
Avrahami, Einat, 1963–
The invading body : reading illness autobiographies / Einat Avrahami.
p.   cm.
Includes bibliographical references and index.
ISBN 978-0-8139-2664-3 (cloth : alk. paper) — ISBN 978-0-8139-2665-0 (pbk. : alk. paper)
1. Terminally ill—Psychology. 2. Terminally ill—Biography. 3. Critically ill—Psychology.
4. Critically ill—Biography. I. Title.
R726.8.A97 2007
610.73'6—dc22
2007010403

FOR TOMER, WITH LOVE

CONTENTS

ACKNOWLEDGMENTS

This work would not have been carried out without the unwavering support of my husband, Tomer Ben Efraim, who helped me in multiple ways, ranging from hunting for illness photographs in downtown Manhattan galleries and looking up reviews of illness memoirs, to taking care of our two children on numerous school vacations and boosting my confidence in moments of despair. I was fortunate to have wise and attentive readers during all the stages of writing this book and to engage in conversations that helped me improve the manuscript. I am very grateful to Ellen Spolsky for her illuminating and sensitive guidance during my early stages of thinking and writing at the University of Bar-Ilan. Special thanks are due to Elana Gomel, Shlomit Rimmon-Kenan, Rachel Salmon, Millette Shamir, and Hana Wirth-Nesher—as well as to the two readers for the University of Virginia Press, one anonymous and the other Ross Chambers—for their generous and perceptive comments on the manuscript. An honorary salute goes to Irma Klein and Edna Rosenthal for their encouragement along the way. I thank Cathie Brettschneider, my editor at the University of Virginia Press, and Beth Ina, freelance copyeditor, for their support and conscientiousness. I'm indebted to James Phelan and Rita Charon for publishing chapters 1 and 3, respectively, in *Narrative* and *Literature and Medicine,* and for the permission to reprint. Gracious permissions to reproduce photographic images, as well as much-needed technical help, were given to me by Terry Dennett at the Jo Spence Archive in London, The Ronald Feldman Fine Arts gallery in New York, the photographer Art Myers, and the artist and photographer Ariela Shavid. I take this opportunity to thank Terry Dennett for bringing to my attention and kindly mailing to me photocopies of the majority of unpublished documents and images relevant to Spence's work with illness and self-representation. Our intense e-mail correspondence during the months I was writing chapter 4 has been an invaluable and edifying resource for clarifying my thought on Spence's various methods of self-documentation and photographic production.

Last but not least, I thank my father, Zvi Avrahami, whose courageous struggle with Parkinson's disease fills me with awe and fortifies my belief that serious illness should be addressed as part of what makes us human. I am equally grateful to my mother, Shoshana Avrahami, whose admirable performance of the caretaking role testifies to the embodied dimension of intersubjectivity and is a steady source of inspiration and relief.

An earlier version of chapter 1, titled "'Keep Your Mind in Hell and Despair Not': Illness as Life Affair in Gillian Rose's *Love's Work*," was published in *Narrative* 9.3 (2001): 305–21. Chapter 3 was published as an essay entitled "Impacts of Truth(s): The Confessional Mode in Harold Brodkey's Illness autobiography" in *Literature and Medicine* 22.2 (2003): 164–87. I am grateful to the publishers for permission to reprint the work here.

THE INVADING BODY

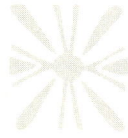

INTRODUCTION: HOW THE "I"
HANDLES FINITENESS

FEW THEORETICAL CONCEPTS SEEM AS HAPPILY RESOLVED AS the fictive nature of the autobiographical self. The critical practice since the late 1970s has been to undermine the belief in the referential relationship between self-representation and lived experience. Autobiography's aspirations to factuality and originality were exposed as false and were promptly discarded by deconstructivists, cultural constructivists, and poststructuralists alike. This rare moment of critical accord is disrupted, however, by the flourishing subgenre of illness autobiographies. Personal narratives of terminal illness stand alone in the world of self-writing since they have the power to question the prevalent descriptions of the category of autobiography as always already created and absorbed by existing cultural constructs and discursive practices. These shocking self-disclosures of symptoms, disabilities, and the uncontrollable physical and psychological pains of treatment, especially when combined with thoughts of further deterioration and of imminent death, are inextricable from the writers' lived experience. Such acts of self-representation are anchored in the occasion of writing to the extent that the writers' very ability to write as well as the meaning of their narratives continue to be contingent on extratextual embodied conditions, as is most dramatically grasped by the readers when they learn of the death of the author.

Autobiographies of people with terminal illness are interesting not only because they problematize the prevailing descriptions of the relationship between lived experience and representation but also because they enact one of the most passionately debated issues in the humanities today: the relationship between subjectivity and the body. Theories of embodiment and of the means by which the materiality of the body is produced have commanded the frontline of research in feminist and cultural studies in the last decade. Pitted against the domineering epistemology and practice of the natural sciences, these theories have reclaimed the body from Cartesian binary thinking and from the model of the body as machine, and celebrated corporeality as "the very 'stuff' of subjectivity" (Grosz, *Volatile Bodies* ix). Surprisingly, however, autobiographical studies—the most obvious locus for testing such theoretical formulations—lags behind contemporary inquiries into the embodied self. Whereas race, gender, and ethnicity are commonplace topics in autobiographical research, the categories of the lived body and of somatic identity have been consigned, to a large extent, to the realm of what has come to be known as disability studies.

Without necessarily referring to the literature on embodiment theory, scholars who write on disability, such as Nancy Mairs, Robert F. Murphy, Lennard J. Davis, and Tobin Siebers, are clearly aware of the disabled body as a dimension of knowledge about the world.[1] They map out "the body" not just as socially constructed, and not just as performing an identity, but also as *phenomenologically* abled in different and decisive ways. Obviously, in the case of the disabled, political affiliations may stem from corporeality. Yet this is also true of the able-bodied. Writers in disability studies tell us that embodied identity in general is not simply an ideological construction: "The disabled body is no more real than the able body—and no less real," says Siebers (749). To put it more boldly, these writers understand that our bodily conditions are often the source of our individual sense of self, even though this conclusion seems to run counter to the logic of much current thought on the fundamentally cultural construction of our identities and our bodies.

Transferring these concerns to the field of autobiography studies must also take into account issues of representation. It is one thing to argue about the formative physical experience of the sick and disabled and an altogether different effort to show how the experience of illness and disability can be rendered. This book is a study of the challenges posed to autobiographical studies as well as to poststructuralist theories of representation by autobiographies that chronicle serious and life-threatening illness. It investigates an array of autobiographical testimonies of terminal illness, including memoirs, journals, photographed self-portraits, and autobiographical essays, with the twofold purpose of, first, advancing critical perception beyond its inability to distinguish between autobiography and fiction and, second, showing the shortcomings of the current theoretical formulations of the body when applied to narrated and photographed concrete cases of collapsed somatic identity.

I approach somatic identity through the contingent and contiguous relationships between writers and artists' experience of terminal illness and their textually or visually displayed selves. Autobiographies of people with terminal illness, I argue, place both their creators and their audience at the intersection of the body and interpretation in a manner that inserts an element of contiguity between the material fatality of physical disease and the cultural construction of illness by discursive practices. The audience thus encounters explorations of the embodiment of the self through both the writer-artist's interpretation of the past and their projection of a future self onto the text. Such acts of projection and reconstruction also inform the processes of reading and viewing, where the audience not only reinterprets the ways in which bodily deterioration mediates someone else's identity but is also led to identify with the writer or artist by projecting their own somatic selves. Whereas today's discursively oriented theory fails to account for this element of contiguity, this study aims to highlight the role of extratextual embodied experience both in constructing these narratives and photographs and in compelling the audience to engage in the multiple-bodied "invasion of the real."

By "invasion of the real," I mean something beyond the closed, formalistic system of narrative patterns and external to the constitutive, nonreferential system of medical practice and cultural myth. It is the experience of illness as a process of learning that underscores the changed body as a source of knowledge. Such lived experience demands to be articulated in language and yet it also defies discursivity, the normative construction of the body. Not surprisingly, then, these texts and images produce a tension between socially constructed materiality and the concrete and idiosyncratic experience of terminal illness that reveals the inadequacy of the available, shared constructs to encompass the range of experiential embodiment.[2]

This is not to say that readers and viewers of illness narratives and photographs encounter lived experience only in terms of the inexpressible. One of Elaine Scarry's insights about the isolation of individuals in pain emphasizes the asymmetry of access to the experiential knowledge that pain dictates: "[T]o have great pain is to have certainty; to hear that another person has pain is to have doubt" (7). Yet, in contrast to Scarry's experiential imbalance, which, ironically, is cast in epistemological terms, my claim is that the confrontation with personal testimonies of illness does not waiver exclusively between the boundaries of cognition, confined to the epistemological poles of certainty and doubt, but creates ethical and emotional engagement in a way that affords something beyond a sense of the indeterminacy of meaning. This is why I wish to accent the gradient of experience begotten through the collaborative processes of writing-photographing and reading-viewing. Such emphasis is crucial to my perception of illness autobiographies not as reproductions of cultural narratives of illness or as dubious stories that the healthy cannot share but rather as sites where cultural narratives intersect with the ways illness is phenomenologically experienced.

The following poem, "Self-Analysis," by Portugal's major twentieth-century writer Fernando Pessoa, illustrates the kind of emotional and ethical engagement that autobiographies of people with terminal illness demand from the audience. Here, the urgency we often associate with the need to empathize with suffering is juxtaposed at once with the poet's rhetorical estrangement from his own pain and with the audience's twice-removed interpretive refashioning of the original experience. The poem suggests that while accurately representing the experience of pain is impossible, readers can still engage in an ethical response to the work by identifying with the voice of an Other in pain through projecting their own map of pain.

> The poet is a forger who
> Forges so completely that
> He forges even the feeling
> He feels as pain.
>
> And those who read his poems
> Feel absolutely, not his two
> Separate pains, but only the
> Pain that they do not feel.
>
> And thus, diverting the
> Understanding, the wind-up
> Train we call the heart
> Runs along its track.

The poet, and by implication all users of language, is "a forger," both a creator and a falsifier; his inscribed experience misrepresents even the most acutely felt pain. However, while the act of writing irrevocably splits the original feeling of pain in two—the "truly" felt and lost pain and the "forged" pain that language constructs—the act of reading unifies the two through a complete substitution of otherness for absence: the readers "Feel absolutely . . . only the / Pain that they do not feel." At once enfolded in the readers' response is an epistemological sense of absence, the pain of unfeeling, and, to my mind, the more intriguing experience of being so completely barred by the impasse of language that they are diverted to a realm external to language, outside the cognitive patterns the poem identifies as "the / Understanding." There, in what for Pessoa constitutes "the heart," readers are forced to defy cognition and accept an emotionally paradoxical stance where they feel only what "they do not feel." So, in a way, the poet's linguistic "forgery" allows the reader to experience what language cannot communicate.

The poem's design of a chain of cognitively inadequate substitutions, in which writing one's pain becomes a misnomer and fabrication enables readers to recognize an Other, is paradigmatic, for Pessoa, of the working of "the wind-up / Train we call the heart." This is not only an abstract claim but one that can be enacted in the process of reading. In other words, the poet's ability to engage the audience in identification through projection adds an emotional dimension more powerful than cognition, or the "Understanding," which is too easily "divert[ed]." Thus, rather than mourn the absence of "genuine" feeling (the original pain) and the loss, furthermore, of the possibility of poetic mimesis, the poem underscores the paradoxically productive emotional dynamics of reading and writing. The process that culminates in readers' feeling "the / Pain that they do not feel" parallels the poet's own process of writing: both reading and writing are depicted as an imaginative embrace of one's projected pain. Sharing the inexpressible becomes possible in spite of the pervasive irony of the attempt, which, diverting intentionality and cognition, proceeds in a spiral-like motion to introduce the audience to an experiential zone that can never be explicitly rendered in the text.

Pessoa's "Self-Analysis" suggests a mode of relating to a wide range of autobiographical testimonies. However, the qualitative difference between autobiographies in general and autobiographies of people with terminal illness is that the latter compel their audience to confront the authors' as well as their own finality. Subsequently, the collaborative effort that they demand from the audience is always subject to empirical reality, even as this reality is consciously manipulated or diverted toward an artistic representation of the autobiographical "I." Illness narratives have been fittingly characterized as "heightening one's awareness of one's mortality, threatening one's sense of identity, and disrupting the apparent plot of one's life" (Couser, *Recovering Bodies* 5). In the current ideological climate, which holds the "fictive nature of selfhood" to be "a biographical fact" (Eakin, *Fictions in Autobiography* 182), it is not unusual to conceive of one's life in terms of a "plot"; indeed, some illness narratives resemble other contemporary forms of autobiography in consciously grappling with modernity's deconstruction of the referential basis of language and, consequently, also with the problematic of moving beyond the text to a knowledge of the self and its world. Yet, far more than any other autobiographical discourse, these narratives are uniquely oriented toward the relationship between lived experience and the textually displayed self.

Writing about one's physical disease ineluctably engages the writer in the real, while reading self-disclosures of the lived experience of illness at once implicates the reader in her own mortality and aims to obliterate the distance between the writer, the text, and the reader. Illness narratives, thus, insert themselves between the referential, "extratextual" reality of the sick writers and the ideological and linguistic constructs of their illness. They do so not because they manage to establish a simple and direct link between the text and the experience of suffering "out there" but because they create a sense of imaginative identification so powerful that its effect is to point the reader outside the text.[3] Thus the truth-value of writing about one's illness emerges from what becomes experience in the process of the telling and its reception,[4] as writers and readers are initiated into an extratextual zone and acknowledge the literal, material basis of the narrative.

Not surprisingly, emerging research in the field of illness narratives, or "pathography" as it has come to be called,[5] has noted the inadequacy of the current skepticism toward the ontology of the autobiographical self in a discussion of writing about one's illness. "In narratives describing illness and death," says Ann Hunsaker Hawkins, "the reader is repeatedly confronted with the pragmatic reality and experiential unity of the autobiographical self" (17). Furthermore,

> Pathography challenges the skepticism of critics and theorists about the self, making that skepticism seem artificial, mandarin, and contrived. The self of pathographical writing is the self-in-crisis: when confronted with serious and life-threatening illness, those possibilities, fictions, metaphors, and versions of self are contracted into a "hard" defensive ontological reality—primed for action, readied for response to the threat of the body, alternatively resisting and inviting the eventual disintegration of the self that is death (Hawkins 17).[6]

In spite of their obvious rhetorical context, illness narratives possess a degree of actuality that compels a connection—for writers and readers— between the author and the narrating self.[7] If autobiography in general, as Philippe Lejeune suggests, can be defined as "a historically variable *contractual effect*" (*On Autobiography* 30), the contract foregrounded by illness narratives requires the reader's full belief in the writer's reality of suffering. Indeed, illness narratives endorse and enact Richard Rorty's notion of "human solidarity . . . based on a [shared] sense of a common danger" (91) by urging readers to imaginatively reconstruct their own future selves as "citizens" of the planet of the sick.[8]

Clearly, however, these narratives exemplify the prevalent critical position in autobiographical studies, which sees writing about one's past as constructed, reordered, and recreated in the process of writing (Hawkins 18). As Scarry has claimed in her groundbreaking study, pain is by definition incommunicable—not simply resisting language but actively destroying it (7). A writer's endeavor to present the trials of illness must therefore take place in episodes of remission, when one is strong enough to recollect and, inevitably, reconstruct the experience of suffering. Arthur W. Frank has this position in mind when he disputes the notion that, since illness narratives are necessarily constructed and often edited, the truth of the personal experience they bear must be questionable: "[E]ven edited stories remain true. The truth of [illness] stories is not only what *was* experienced, but equally what *becomes* experience in the telling and its reception" (22). Yet, granted that illness narratives do not simply record but rather reconstruct the experience of illness, how are we to reconcile our awareness of their conventional literariness with the opposite intuitive reception of these texts as authentic records of individual suffering? How do such narratives compel our collaboration in rendering the body articulate, and, as Couser has put it, how do they "foreground somatic experience in a new way by treating the body's form and function (apart from race or gender) as fundamental constituents of identity" (*Recovering Bodies* 12)?

What I call the "reality effect" of illness narratives has to do with the unsettling tension they sustain between the writers' appropriation of their experience through language and the materiality of the physical transformation they speak of, where the lived body takes over, undergoing uncontrolled changes that are obviously undesired and unwelcome. The felt tension between empowerment and powerlessness points to the invasion of the text by the sick body. Insistently, the reader is directed toward the extratextual occasion of writing and is asked to confront the limitations and shared risks of mortality. Illness narratives, therefore, enact a movement from materiality to construction that occurs when one's body suddenly grows out of step with one's psyche. Not only in terms of motivation for writing but also within the texts themselves, the body's "fall" out of categories of normalcy instigates the writers' and readers' reevaluation of the relationship between the discursive and the real.

The relationship between lived experience and its representations has been, of course, a cardinal concern for autobiographical studies in the last decades. While the dominant trend in autobiographical studies today has been to dispense with the concept of the self as transcendent and autonomous and concede its contingent and provisional nature, the enduring controversy bears heavily on the contested status of autobiography as either a distinct genre or a series of narrative arrangements that are indistinguishable from fiction. In general terms, the debate opposes those who mourn the illusiveness of the aspiration of autobiography to move beyond its own text to a knowledge of the self and its world, to others, whose understanding that the self displays rather than distorts itself by means of language has led to new perspectives about the relationship between the autobiographical text and lived experience.[9]

Theories of deconstruction strongly influenced the skeptical approach of the first wave of poststructuralist critics in autobiographical studies, whose aim was to question the mimetic relation between textual representation and lived experience. Throughout the 1980s, the critical bon ton was to treat the truth of the autobiographical "I" as discursively determined and therefore fictitious.[10] In his 1980 introduction to *Autobiography: Essays Theoretical and Critical,* James Olney aptly summed up the direction taken in the late 1970s by poststructuralist and deconstructionist critics who focused on the epistemological impasses that stemmed from the collapse of the formerly stable elements of history and subjectivity in one's personal story, the *bios* and *autos* of an autobiography. These critics, says Olney, have demonstrated that the autobiographical text "takes a life of its own, and the self that was not really in existence in the beginning is in the end merely a matter of text and has nothing to do with an authorizing author. The self [*autos*], then, is a fiction and so is the life [*bios*], and behind the text of an autobiography lies the text of an 'autobiography': all that is left are characters on a page and they too can be 'deconstructed' to demonstrate the shadowiness of even their existence" (22).

Nevertheless, autobiography continues to elicit intense critical interest in respect to the politics of writing in the first person, the historically dynamic mechanisms of genre formation, and the exploration of the conflicting and contested racial, class, and gender discursive fields that produce and in turn are affected by personal and collective identities. What distinguishes the current generation of critics in autobiographical studies from the earlier poststructuralist critics is that they, and particularly the feminist and postcolonialist critics among them, assume from the start that the subject of autobiography is "necessarily discursive" (Gilmore, "Mark of Autobiography" 3). This conceptual vantage point has enabled contemporary scholars to (re)describe autobiography as a distinct genre. Following Foucault, they have traced the origin and evidential force of autobiographical texts to the historical evolution of political, culturally bound conditions and values that have constituted self-writing as a discourse of truth. Accordingly, the autobiographical text "draws its social authority from its relation to culturally dominant discourses of truthtelling and not, as has previously been asserted, from autobiography's privileged relation to real life" (Gilmore, "Mark" 9). One of the major consequences, then, of the poststructuralist attempt to theorize the subject as constituted in discourse has been the reopening of the relationship between text and context insofar as identities produced in texts—like identities in "real life"—are agreed to be subjected to regulatory discursivity. Cultural constructivism, joined with weaker poststructuralist formulations of the political and symbolic interactions among social groups, has provided the theoretical underpinnings for viewing identity—in autobiography and in life—as "discursive, provisional, intersectional, and unfixed" (Smith and Watson 20).

My own reading of personal accounts of illness also acknowledges them as invariably anchored in and shaped by the dominant cultural discourses that produce the medical truths or meanings of certain illnesses. Such testimonial acts occur in a social world in which the ill possess a recognized status and where cultural institutions and social practices not only regulate lived experience but have performative functions with regard to the individual's endeavor to describe his or her experience of suffering. A network of discourses, moreover, constitutes the social relations of power that produce the identity and cultural marginalization of the ill. These cultural forces mediate the experiences of sickness and death and in turn affect our deepest anxieties in respect to terminal illness. As Treya Killam Wilber's cancer journal makes clear, a patient's experience is by no means restricted to the constructs produced by the medical system: "A cloud of voices, images, ideas, fears, stories, photographs, advertisements, articles, movies, television shows arises around me, vague, shapeless, but dense, ominous. These are the stories my culture has collected around this thing, 'the big C'" (38). Surely, the meeting ground between writers and readers of illness autobiographies is better illuminated by approaches more attentive to social and historical discursive conditions than to the deconstructive vision of language as an impersonal and autonomous system.

And yet, as this study will also show, even the weaker formulations of cultural constructionism fail to account for the ways illness autobiographies juxtapose cultural constructs such as the "truth" of breast cancer, say, or the "identity" of a person with AIDS, with the historically specific, socially and physiologically concrete experience of individual embodiment.[11] As a way of interpreting autobiographical testimonies of illness, that is, cultural constructionism shares with deconstruction a tendency to objectify somatic identity as the subject of inquiry, to position, in Bruce R. Smith's words, "the analyst here and *it* over there so that it can be seen, known, mastered" (325). For the deconstructivists' maintenance of "a secure vantage point in language that leads to [discursive] aporia" (Smith 325), constructionist readings substitute a no less purportedly secure political vantage point that highlights relations of power as the constant (if formally variegated and historically dynamic) forces behind meaning-making linguistic structures and social institutions. Illness autobiographies, in contrast, disclose the crucial role of bodily transformation in self-examination and self-reconstruction practices. They insist on the concretely situated body not only as an undeniable reality that should be reckoned with but also as an indispensable source of knowledge, stressing the experience of terminal illness as an embodied process of learning to live with extreme physiological, and not merely social, constraints. Granted that cultural constructs do shape the experience and behavior of the sick, so too does the materiality of bodily transformation and deterioration, where lived experience becomes contingent on somatic, rather than wholly cultural, limitations.

It is in the wake of this critical shift from Foucauldian political readings to more recent understandings of the embodiment of the self that I place my claim to the unique status of illness autobiographies.[12] Terminal illness narratives and photographs alert us to the problems that arise from treating historically specific bodies as textual, and rather passive, surfaces whose meaning is determined by social institutions and discourses. They question the prevailing poststructuralist perspective that has generated neat formulations of materiality, and of the body, as always already a discursive construct, the product of conscious or unconscious political inscription. A leading argument in poststructuralist feminist theory, eloquently presented by Judith Butler in her 1993 book *Bodies That Matter,* is that not only gender, or even sex, but indeed the materiality of the body itself is a construct produced by cultural discourses that serve to promote the system's heterosexual imperatives. In other words, Butler traces a movement from construction to materialization, where the body stands as the constituted effect of a matrix of gender relations. Illness autobiographies, however, challenge this view of the body as a secondary product of the normative discursive system. They highlight, instead, the interrelatedness and interconstitutive dynamics of embodied experience and discursive constructs. Such a dynamics is established on the phenomenological and cognitive tension between the already known and the drastically changed circumstances of a lived body that can no longer be accommodated by past experience and therefore demands openness to new embodied knowledge. This is not to deny that the prevalent idea that "bodies . . . are not born; they are made" (Haraway 207) has greatly contributed to our understanding of the body as the result of a historical and cultural process of materialization which, as feminist critics have shown, can be channeled to diverse political uses. Still, the illness autobiographies examined in this book demonstrate that neat theoretical formulations of materiality cannot accommodate the messy reality of the lived body.

THE INVADING BODY

It is here that my interest in illness autobiographies converges with more general contemporary attempts to theorize the embodied subject. However, whereas theory almost by definition depends on broad and inclusive concepts, personal accounts of illness insist on the explanatory power of particular cases. My analysis of these accounts thus follows Toril Moi's injunction to view the concrete example not as a secondary illustration of a general rule but as "the place where thought happens, where theoretical questions get raised, elaborated, and answered" (302). Too often in the current research on the body, the concrete case is relegated to a secondary place in favor of more comprehensive theoretical formulations. Thus, even Elizabeth Grosz, whose enormous contribution to theories of the body is unquestionable, concedes the "ability of bodies to always extend the frameworks which attempt to contain them" (xi) only to strive, at the same time, to rethink the body in terms of a general great theory. As the title of her 1994 book attests, *Volatile Bodies: Toward a Corporeal Feminism* is an ambitious endeavor to reconcile incongruous theories, including phenomenological, psychoanalytical, and sociopolitical readings of the body, through the suggestive image of Lacan's Möbius strip (xii). "Bodies," Grosz proposes, "have all the explanatory power of minds"; therefore, "all the effects of subjectivity, all the significant facets and complexities of subjects, can be as adequately explained using the subject's corporeality as a framework as it would be using consciousness or the unconscious" (vii). And yet, as she also admits, what her book presents is "a series of disparate, indeed kaleidoscopic and possibly contradictory" theories and ideas (xiv).

Illness autobiographies are illuminating precisely because they enact one of the major obstacles in the attempt to reconcile the current frameworks that contain the body, for they grapple—urgently and pragmatically—with the felt incongruity between the culturally tractable body and the experientially unruly and yet constraining body. As Drew Leder has observed, most of the dominant approaches to the subject's embodiment in the twentieth century fall under two primarily conflicting registers, which he terms "the phenomenological" and "the sociopolitical" ("Introduction" 4). In brief, the phenomenological register, which roughly corresponds to "the inside out" in Grosz's terminology, focuses on the ways our experiencing and experienced bodies beget our worlds, including our consciousness, language, and social interactions. The sociopolitical approach—Grosz's "the outside in"—reads bodies as malleable surfaces whose diverse meanings are inscribed by powerful social and political discursive practices. Because of the promise it offers for ideological and social transformation, and probably also because of fortuitous historical and political conditions within the academic world, the "malleable body" approach is today undoubtedly the more influential of the two. For very similar reasons, in autobiographical studies, much as in cultural and feminist studies, the sociopolitical approach to issues of identity and subject-formation prevails. While illness autobiographies do not finally resolve the problem by presenting an orderly and unified concept of embodiment, they nonetheless underline the uneasy coexistence of the lived body with the multiply inscribed cultural body and emphasize the need to attend to experiential accounts of illness on their own messy terms.

This seemingly modest demand has far-reaching significance in respect to recognizing the distinctiveness of illness narratives and photographs within the category of self-representation. Writers and photographers of illness testimonies establish their authority by using the phenomenological leverage they have gained in the transition from occupying the unmarked status of healthy bodies to being identified and identifying themselves with the drastically reduced position of the sick. This unusual vantage point mobilizes their accounts of illness as a complex experiential amalgam of cultural constructs, political inscriptions, and uncontrollable physiological processes that ultimately defy discursivity. While the current critical view in autobiographical studies traces the truth-value of autobiography to social and institutional discourses of truth-telling, illness autobiographies pull us back to the confrontation with the idiosyncratic validity and veracity of concretely situated, embodied experiences.

By underscoring the very real consequences, for the authors, of physiological, organic, and biological processes both at the present time of production and in the future, when their texts-works will be read, illness narratives and photographs anticipate and shape the reaction of their audience. Accordingly, the audience's interactions with these texts are both embodied and rhetorical. The felt demand with which illness narratives and photographs address their audience—that of sustaining an awareness of the corporeal significance and extratextual consequences of the represented events—distinguishes this subgenre from other modes of autobiographical performance. At once complying with, and yet resisting, the current description of autobiography as a nonreferential genre of self-representation, internally organized by norms and narrative patterns and externally provided with a cultural stamp of truth, illness autobiographies emerge as a nonfocal member at the boundaries of "autobiography" as a category.[13] Once we acknowledge that illness autobiographies are defined by their unique relationship of contiguity and contingency with extratextual reality, we cannot easily cling to a description that identifies autobiography directly with the discursive attributes of its most representative exemplars. Even though, operationally, we can continue to evaluate "autobiography" through its clearest cases, the presence of the subgenre of illness autobiographies at the fuzzy edge of the category problematizes accepted definitions of the category.

Yet, the shift from the prevailing sociopolitical critique to a criticism that aspires to account also for the lived, experienced, and experiencing body is not an easy move. In discussions of this book with respectable academics from the humanities, I was asked again and again to provide tangible proof for the existence of terminal illness in the text. "How can it be," people asked, "that illness autobiographies and photographs contain contiguous relationships with extratextual reality? How can the sick body 'really' enter the image or the text?" "Well," I would usually attempt to answer, "of course there is no *blood* in the text, but the experience of serious illness elicits certain kinds of new embodied knowledge." "In that case," my interlocutors would respond, "why should this be any different for the more normative autobiographies?" My answer to these critics is that there should not be a difference in theory, but that in practice, the few critical attempts to wrestle with the concept of embodiment in autobiographical studies have not proven helpful in clarifying their own terms. Too often, the concept of the embodied subject is thrown in as one of the criteria of the autobiographical narrative in a manner that comes close to paying lip service to current theoretical fashion. Thus, "the body" has been recently defined as "a site of autobiographical knowledge because memory itself is embodied," while "life narratives" are taken for granted, tautologically, as "sites of embodied knowledge because autobiographical narrators are embodied subjects" (Smith and Watson 21). Such an approach reveals the limitation of strong prescriptive categories that remain untested by particular examples. By contrast, the texts and images I examine are concrete test cases of autobiographical work that elicit, on the one hand, the controversy in autobiographical studies over issues of self-representation and self-invention and that enact, on the other hand, the exclusionary as well as the intercorporeal processes by which the materiality of the body is produced.

The following discussion of specific illness autobiographies and photographed self-portraits, then, investigates the special and the conventional attributes that constitute the borderline locale of this subgenre in respect to the autobiographical prototype. As was suggested by my initial discussion of the topic, this book draws on a wide range of methodological resources that are not always easily distinguishable from "theory." These include contemporary phenomenological readings of the lived body influenced by Paul Schilder and Maurice Merleau-Ponty; cultural studies of medical history and of the social significance of certain illnesses; feminist and deconstructive studies of the ontological status of the embodied subject; and insights gleaned from late twentieth-century semiotic and poststructuralist inquiries into photography's reality effect and evidential force. In addition, I embrace the implicit guidelines for reading presented by the autobiographical texts themselves, some of which are in fact academic essays and others of which are written by established writers and scholars. Using these various resources has been in accord with my interdisciplinary approach to illness narratives and photographs both as literary and cultural products and as speech acts and visual performances that demand for the teller and actor the status of an active agent. At the same time, I am interested in the collaborative rhetorical effort of writers and readers, photographers and viewers, as a means of clearing a viable place for an empathic and ethical response to the experience of illness and to the ill as fully fledged subjects rather than as objects of pity.

To pursue this book's twin goals—to provide an account of the unique status of illness autobiographies and to acknowledge the idiosyncratic

THE INVADING BODY

ethical and cultural work they do—each chapter places in dialogue personal illness narratives with critical and theoretical discourses on illness and self-representation. Chapter 1, "Illness as Life Affair in Gillian Rose's *Love's Work*," examines Gillian Rose's much-praised illness autobiography, *Love's Work: A Reckoning with Life*, from a narratological perspective. It begins by placing Rose's text within the larger context of this growing genre, working against the claims of critics who assume that illness narratives are not just cultural constructs but predictable constructs doggedly employing conventional narrative devices and conforming to prevalent cultural myths.[14] While all of the writers and photographers whose work I discuss demonstrate and even foreground, through conscious references and refashioning, their awareness of their own appropriation by cultural identities, Rose's autobiography is the most powerful test case for "the invasion of the real" that I find characteristic of many illness stories. As a professor of modern philosophy, Rose is acutely aware of modernity's crises of interpretation. Her autobiography presents a writer's conscious grappling with the act of telling her story, and it is a mesmerizing voyage into the complexity of representation. Rose's struggle to represent her experience of illness is at once cognitive and emotive, but most of all, it is bodily, highlighting the contiguity between illness and language. Her text also illustrates the specificity of illness autobiographies' demand for rhetorical collaboration with their audiences. My analysis of her narrative is an attempt to enact what it means to engage in reading illness autobiographies on their own terms.

Chapter 2, "First You Hurt," moves from the narratological framework used in chapter 1 to a phenomenological approach to sick selves. Here, I examine the most distinctive attribute of illness autobiographies: their representation not just of a self but, crucially, of an embodied self. This chapter provides new readings of breast-cancer journals, memoirs, and autobiographical essays, including Audre Lorde's well-known *The Cancer Journals*, Eve Kosofsky Sedgwick's essay "White Glasses," and less familiar but no less resonant memoirs by Musa Mayer, Christina Middlebrook, Treya Killam Wilber, and Barbara Rosenblum. My choice to discuss personal accounts of breast cancer is not arbitrary, particularly in light of the normative construction of breasts in Western patriarchy as the supreme visual mark of femininity. Breast-cancer journals provide rich phenomenological resources for studying the interaction between gendered and somatic identities as well as for testing poststructuralist and feminist descriptions of the cultural source of embodied states and processes. Focusing first on Lorde's and Mayer's cancer memoirs in the context of the prevailing feminist discourses on breast reconstruction and cosmetic surgery, the chapter then turns to the other authors' endeavors to demetaphorize their struggle with metastatic, indeed terminal, breast cancer. Like Rose's *Love's Work,* the latter texts demonstrate that the traditional divisions between the cultural and the somatic cannot accommodate the reality of living with illness. At the same time, as the chapter suggests, illness narratives' perception of the lived body as a source of knowledge can advance feminist theory and feminist politics of transformation beyond the reductive scope of the essence/construction debate.

Chapter 3, "Confessing AIDS," juxtaposes my argument about terminal illness as a mode of learning with an ethical inquiry into the mechanisms of strong constructionism, which seriously impoverishes our understanding of illness narratives and the experience of coming to terms with illness. The chapter offers a revision of the influential Foucauldian conception of the power relations inherent in autobiography and tests its applicability to illness narratives by distinguishing between recollection of the sick body as a textual construction and recollection as embodied experience. The first part of the discussion highlights the ways structural and thematic elements of autobiographical discourse intersect with the dominant cultural narratives of terminal illness and, thus, serve to reinforce the interpellation of the ill as abject bodies and social outcasts. However, in the second part of the discussion, the role of embodied experience as a source of knowledge is developed through a close reading of Harold Brodkey's illness autobiography *This Wild Darkness: The Story of My Death.* Brodkey's compelling example enacts the interrelationship between textual and cultural practices in illness autobiographies, and yet it also shows how narratives of illness enable writers to recall the sick body not only as a textual and cultural construction but in terms of embodied, embedded experience. Over and against the power of cultural constructs to produce a recollection of the body as textuality, my reading underlines

Brodkey's achievement in articulating the sick body as material and inter-corporeal agency. In spite of its sophistication and literary finesse, Brod-key's book has so far attracted scant critical attention—an unfortunate oversight that this chapter attempts to rectify.

The next two chapters transport the analysis of embodied recollection from self-writing to self-photographing and are best read as one theo-retical unit. Chapters 4 and 5 propose that the self-reflexive gaze at the sick body has the power to question current theoretical tenets about the medium of photography as textuality. They identify autobiographical illness photographs as an emerging subgenre of self-documentation whose indexical relationship with the reality of illness parallels the conti-guity of illness narratives with somatic experience. Chapter 4, "Flesh-tinted Frames," focuses on the gradient of indexicality in Jo Spence's au-tobiographical illness photographs, explored through the processes of their production and reception. Arguing against structuralist and post-structuralist assumptions of a clear-cut separation of photographic rep-resentation from prephotographic reality, the chapter shows that the tes-timonial force of these photographs is better explained by attending to the dynamic processes of photographic production and reception that shift the evidential force of photography from the subject of the image to the viewer's sense of time. Exploring this shift is especially productive in examining the unique power of illness photographs to embrace both our understanding of their coded messages and our incongruent notion that the suffering they convey is real—not only in the sense that "this is how it was" but also in grasping that the time elapsed since a given photograph was made matters crucially to the people who are photographed.

The close analysis of Spence's illness photographs serves as a model for studying the range of the relation between construction and contiguity, the function of which is tested in the last chapter, "Hannah Wilke: Per-forming Grief." This chapter discusses Hannah Wilke's 1992 *Intra-Venus* cancer photographs in terms of their ongoing vacillation between the boundaries of construction and contiguity. Placed in the context of Wilke's lifelong engagement in performance art, the discussion first ex-amines her cancer photographs' testimonial and ethical work in juxta-posing conventional cultural icons with metonymic invocations of the her own sick body. Later on, the analysis of her more direct confrontation with illness emphasizes the difference between her extremely disturbing chemotherapy self-portraits and other contemporary photographed representations of triumphantly recovered bodies. Unlike the other photographs, Wilke's photographs do powerful performative work in shocking the audience into a recognition of moral and rhetorical complicity. Our guilty awareness of being moved by her art at the expense of her life pulls our attention away from the deliberately symbolic, contrived, and manipulated meanings and balances them against a sense of real consequences beyond the photographs' frame. Indeed, Wilke's and Spence's illness photographs are interesting not simply for their staggering visual thematization of the sick body, but because they test the current critical consensus about the medium of photography as wholly manipulated by arbitrary visual signs. They question the logic of the dominant critical claim that, because the reality effect of photographs is necessarily constructed by signs, these signs must have no indexical connection with the reality to which they point. My claim in both of these chapters is that the paradoxical constellation of construction and contiguity, which is the hallmark of even the most postmodern of illness photographs, identifies these photographs as a distinct subgenre of self-documentation. They emerge as nonfocal exemplars within the category of photographic self-representation in ways that parallel the location of illness autobiographies at the fuzzy edge of the category of autobiography.

To identify autobiographical illness narratives and photographs as nonfocal cases that test the current descriptions of the category of self-representation is to emphasize the ongoing interaction and interconstitution of embodied experience and discursive constructs in the situated first-person accounts of historically and socially concrete individuals. These interconstitutive elements are inextricable from the subgenre's unique testimonial force and truth-value. As we shall see, they both condition the specific occasions and acts of writing and photographing and continue to operate at the receiving end of the audience's (re)reading and (re)viewing the texts and photographs.

1

ILLNESS AS LIFE AFFAIR IN
GILLIAN ROSE'S *LOVE'S WORK*

GILLIAN ROSE'S *LOVE'S WORK: A RECKONING WITH LIFE* (1995) IS
an exceptional illness narrative, perhaps because, first and foremost, it is
a masterful autobiography. Intertextually layered, intricate, and thought
provoking, Rose's writing is a self-reflexive attempt to represent the experience of illness as inextricable from and embedded within the values and
contingencies of one's whole life. This position differs drastically from the
usual authorial stance of illness narratives, which seeks to construct a coherent story out of bodily dysfunction (Couser, *Recovering Bodies* 14). Indeed, rather than let the experience of illness serve as the major plot of her
narrative, Rose defers the disclosure of her terminal illness until late in the
book, not revealing it until she has established the thematic concerns and
writer-reader relationship that join her illness story with her complex
view of life. When she does account for the ovarian cancer from which she
had suffered during the process of writing (and of which she died in 1995),
her narrative compresses and even omits major events and typical scenes
of treatment, focusing, rather, on a relatively minor physical condition
through which she articulates the epistemological difficulties, the incompatible choices, and the impasses involved in telling about one's experience of terminal illness. Such a conscious grappling with the act of telling
distinguishes *Love's Work* from the growing body of illness narratives in

England and in the United States. In contrast with the chronological plot, "realistic" setting, and unified narrative voice that govern the majority of personal illness stories, Rose's book strategically interweaves temporalities, locations, and first- and third-person voices as a way of rendering her illness as at once private and common—incommunicable and universally accessible. But to fully understand both why these narrative features are so unusual and how they signify, we need to understand the relation of Rose's narrative to the emerging genre of illness autobiographies.

Collectively viewed, illness narratives tend to be rather formulaic and structurally conventional, manifesting recurrent patterns of plot, closure, audience, and purpose, as well as formative scenes, motifs, and metaphorical paradigms.[1] Commonly, illness autobiographies use the experience of illness as "a turning point around which authors retrospectively interpret their life before the crisis and prospectively plan the life that lies ahead" (Hawkins 37). More commonly, their master plot extends chronologically, from the narrator's detection of a lump or other minor symptoms of the disease, through tests, diagnosis, hospitalization, surgery, chemotherapy, radiation, and partial recovery. Closure, thus, tends to be comic— "the protagonist is better off at the end than at the beginning" (Couser, *Recovering Bodies* 91)—a strategic vantage point that sustains illness narratives' chief purpose of helping others undergoing a similar illness. In illness narratives, "the need to *tell* others so often becomes the wish to *help* others" (Hawkins 25), a motive for writing that invokes a built-in audience of those at risk (Hawkins 33; Couser, *Recovering* 183). These conventional writing patterns have certain beneficial effects for writers and readers alike: "[T]he generic plot provides a convenient narrative armature for the author and a source of predictable gratification for the reader (who is generally assured of the narrator's recovery)" (Couser, *Recovering* 43).[2] Yet, resorting to the familiar formula and the altruistic purpose of addressing others who are ill unwittingly endorses and thereby serves to reinforce the cultural separation of the sick from the healthy.

While illness narratives succeed in posing an alternative to the case report, the genre of medical history written by physicians (Hawkins 12–13), they are less successful in supplanting the prevailing cultural imperative to treat disease as exogenous to the body and, by implication, as alien to

THE INVADING BODY

life itself. This ideological stance is disclosed by the organizing metaphors adopted in the texts, which Hawkins has detected and grouped according to distinct mythical formulations. "Over and over again, the same metaphorical paradigms are repeated in pathographies: the paradigm of regeneration, the idea of illness as battle, the athletic ideal, the journey into a distant country, and the mythos of healthy-mindedness" (27). What these different paradigms share is a Manichean representation of illness as an alien invasion of the healthy body, which can be exorcised or at least held at bay by recourse to several definite strategies. Whether these strategies involve faith in seasonal regeneration, active fighting (as in a battle or a game), going on a quest, or assuming the attitude of healthy-mindedness, illness is ultimately seen as the negation of rather than as an aspect in one's life. Even though these paradigms derive from Western myth and therefore can be said to connect illness stories to storytelling about life at large, the selective ways in which they shape the experience of illness set it as a realm apart from life. When these paradigms are combined with the conventional writing patterns of the genre, they may further reduce the complexity of the experience of illness by assuring the audience of the narrator's personal autonomy, and of her subsequent ability to end her story by leaving the realm of illness safely behind.

Gillian Rose's illness autobiography, by contrast, makes few concessions to the audience. Wary of the reader's need for the familiar, Rose's text consciously isolates itself from the dominant writing and reading conventions provided by the recently flourishing subgenre. Unlike the prevalent pattern in illness narratives, which proceed in a more or less linear fashion, narrating first the author's discovery of being ill, and then the following hardships of treatment, Rose's *Reckoning* seems at first sight to smooth over, ignore, and even belittle the moment of discovery when she finds out that she is ill—and, indeed, her experience of terminal illness. Perhaps this is why the conventional closure that promises the narrator is "healed, if not cured" (Couser, *Recovering* 39), fails to apply to this text: Rose plainly owns that, with or without treatment, she has "less than months of well-being, and, eminently, not years" (102). Yet while she avoids the generic master plot with its inherent constructs of audience and purpose, she uses other narrative strategies to shape her experience of illness and to convey her active involvement both in coming to terms with cancer and in anticipating and directing her audience's response. Thus, she writes an autobiography, not simply an illness story, in which she alternates between the roles of witness and protagonist, negotiating all along her relation to the reader through self-reflexive "wooing" (77) and direct appeal. These narrative choices reflect a clear ideological stance. While the conventional writing patterns of the genre implicitly reiterate the cultural isolation of the sick, Rose wishes to heighten her readers' sensitivity to the dichotomies that sever what she can only experience holistically. Merging her illness with the more inclusive text of her life, her writing strives to redefine terminal illness as an opportunity to understand, as she puts it, "'life' in the meaningful sense, inclusive of death" (79).

Rose's narrative provides a superb test case for "the invasion of the real," the previously identified "reality effect" characteristic of illness stories—not least because, as a professor of modern philosophy, Rose is acutely aware of modernity's crises of interpretation. As I will show, her text is haunted by the desire for linguistic control over both the rendering of her illness and its reception by the reader. The risk of distorting one's private experience of illness is repeatedly presented as succumbing either to an excess of conventional speech or to inarticulate mumbling and silence. Furthermore, the concepts of health and illness themselves are evaluated along the poles of verbal balance and imbalance. In accordance with Scarry's formulation of the experience of pain, health here stipulates command of the individual's capacity for communication, whereas illness threatens to strip the subject of her identity either by silencing or by collapsing the self into ready platitudes and conventional metaphors. Thus, terminal illness, which obviously undermines one's normative control of the body, is shown to be analogous to the rhetoric in which the experience of illness is inscribed. Both in terms of its subject matter and at the level of the telling, the text vacillates between a sense of power and powerlessness as the very attempt to relate to one's illness and thereby constitute its meaning threatens to rob the speaker of her authorial control. As Rose explicitly points out, the rhetorical circumstances of illness narratives ensure that the text is also attacked from without. By invariably invoking in the reader a string of "illness metaphors" and cultural clichés, which in turn are projected onto the text, the writer's control over her experience of illness is again eroded by public speech.

Rose's relational view of the way definitions of illness are negotiated frames the opening of her narrative. Significantly, she begins her autobiography by describing her encounters with seriously ill people, who, moreover, have been or are going to become important agents in her life. These are Edna, whom she soon comes to call her "Intelligent Angel"; Jim, an old and dear friend stricken with AIDS, and Gary, Edna's kind and caring employer. Tellingly situated in the first chapter, these encounters enact a framework for the kind of writer-reader relationship that the narrator will later expect from her own readers, who, like her, become witnesses of illness. In writing about these early encounters, Rose discloses her own initial resistance and "conventionally" horrified reaction to the others' physical and emotional afflictions, but she goes on to tell how she overcame this resistance. In positioning herself as a reader of others' struggles with disease—first as an inadequate, conventional reader, but then as altogether ceasing to "see" the physical signs of sickness—she models for readers how to engage with her own testimony of sickness. The transformative process she enacts cautions against the too-familiar response to the sick as mere objects composed by their symptoms.

By occupying the double role of spectator and agent, Rose further insists that how a person conventionally (which for her is the same thing as "immediately" or "intuitively") views the sickness of others is a very different experience from the way sick people relate to themselves. Accordingly, her third-person descriptions of sickness often exaggerate its perverse and pathological aspects, whereas first-person accounts (including, later, those of her own symptoms) are seldom horrified or horrifying. How you see others, it is implied, is not only very different from how you see yourself but also shaped to a greater extent by fears and cultural boundaries that separate the normal from the pathological. Such a deliberate distinction between the self- and other mode of perception has the converse effect of contributing to one of Rose's major purposes in writing: her desire to reduce the distance between readers and writers of illness narratives, so that witnessing and experiencing illness will not be perceived as unbridgeable modes of being.

That the encounters with her sick friends in the first chapter are integrally related to her writing on her own illness is evident, too, from the strong connections they envisage between illness and language, or, more accurately, between illness and a certain economy of speech. Thematically, these encounters introduce three alternative modes of addressing the relationship between illness and language, all of which reverberate throughout the narrative. The first encounter outlines an urgent, wretched need to make the experience of illness known through continuous and excessive speech that verges on verbal incontinence. The second foregrounds the incommunicability of illness by altogether refusing to acknowledge it in words, and the third posits the need to relearn to speak as a result of severe physical challenge. As the following discussion will show, the opposite positions of telling too much or too little of one's illness are proclaimed inadequate throughout the text, most poignantly when the narrator struggles with her relation to her own illness. Shaped as odd and even perverse, these ways of telling are rejected in favor of acknowledging that illness requires the individual to relearn to speak. Physical trauma may frustrate speech, but it may also instigate a new discourse and, thereby, a new relation to the self. Yet, throughout the narrative, the two rejected modes are not successfully discarded but ever present, threatening to usurp the narrator's sense of self-empowerment and linguistic control.

The risk of losing oneself to verbal incontinence is displayed in the meeting with Jim, whom the narrator has not seen for five years and who has since been identified as HIV-positive. At Newark Airport, where they have arranged to meet, she "first walk[s] up . . . to the wrong man—to someone who looked like a caricature of Jim as I remembered him in good health" (4). But this false recognition does not prevent her from reading into the actual encounter a preconceived conviction about the interchangeability of physical and mental degeneration. When she eventually sees Jim, she observes: "His posture was as crumpled as the clothes he'd obviously slept in, his hair had turned gingerish and it rose from his head in wild clumps with bald patches in between. This uneven growth dominated his manners, too" (4). It soon becomes clear that not only does she compare the sick Jim with the healthy friend she used to know, but that the basis of comparison is a model of normalcy as verbal balance, from which he sadly deviates: "My formerly laconic and witty friend had become loquacious, needy, addressing with urgent familiarity everyone we chanced to have dealings with over the next few days—taxi-drivers, bell-boys, waiters. And when he wasn't holding forth to those nearest to him, he issued a continuous, low, moaning sound, a piteous cradling for the inner, wounded being that, strangely, had surrendered to the publicity of the city streets" (4). The need for linguistic continence and restraint read into Jim's behavior seems to be motivated by the narrator's perception of physical and mental health in terms of social and verbal propriety. Such a perception dictates a pejorative view of illness, since it draws a sharp line between the sick as social transgressors and the healthy as useful members of society. Thus, she says, "I soon learnt to recognize multitudes like [Jim]: the old men in their forties, shrivelled, drained, mumbling across the intersections, icons of AIDS, amidst the bodiful vibrancy of those striding to and from work and subways and stores" (4–5). Bodily "vibrancy," then, is equated not only with a purposeful stride but also with a purposeful speech marked by the absence of "moaning" and "mumbling." Ironically, this dichotomous view of illness and health deprives both the sick and the healthy of their individuality, branding the former as "icons" of disease set against a uniform mass "normality."

The shortcoming of such cultural segregation is soon revealed in the encounters with Gary and Edna, which mark the onset of the narrator's process of education. To her surprise, Gary is "utterly unfazed by Jim's doleful appearance and low-pitched litany" (5), while Edna takes to Jim on first sight, so that even the obtuse narrator cannot but notice, and "not for the last time, the delight that flew between [them]" (8). Themselves seriously ill, Gary and Edna at once help the narrator to correct her conventional, dehumanizing view of illness, and offer two alternative models for enacting the relationship between illness and language. The meeting with Gary, although brief, indicates a relationship by negation, since Gary's sickness, while immediately perceived, is never verbally defined or acknowledged. "I had been told," says the narrator, "that [Gary] was a private scholar, a man of means and intellect, meticulous and courteous. So he was: but I had not been told that he was afflicted with a long-term wasting disease that left him with uneven gait and hands locked in a rictus-like claw" (5). The omission of illness from the descriptions of Gary, and the fact that he does not mention it either when he introduces himself at their meeting, is conceived by the narrator to be "as bizarre in its own way as the first [encounter with Jim]" (5). Still, Gary's "wasting disease" affects neither his manners nor his intellect, and, thus, confutes the narrator's previous equation between illness and mental depravity.

It is with Edna, however, that the "increasingly confused" (6) narrator undergoes a long process of education that causes her to discard her stereotypic response to illness and its relation to language. At the age of ninety-three, Edna has contracted cancer of the face that has not only mutilated her face (her nose had to be removed) but also directly damaged her language skills: "as a result of a prosthetic jaw, [she] had had to relearn to speak" (6). Nonetheless, this predicament seems in no way to restrict Edna's productive life, so much so that she easily fits into the narrator's previous category of normalcy—"the bodiful vibrancy of those striding to and from work and subways and stores" (5). Edna "goes out to work for Gary seven days a week, taking the bus uptown, but often walking the thirty or so blocks back downtown. She acts as Gary's hands, word-processing his scholarship and correspondence" (7). The transgression Edna's illness has committed her to is cosmetic rather than cognitive: her face, distorted by cancer, is "dominated by a false nose, which lacked any cosmetic alleviation whatsoever. Smooth and artificially flesh-coloured, with thick spectacles perched on top, this proboscis could have come from a Christmas cracker" (7). It is only a matter of days, however, before the narrator altogether ceases to see this as an oddity. When Edna inquires whether Rose would mind if she did not put on her nose in the morning, the narrator says: "By then, not only did I not notice the nose, but, if anything, I found the neat, oblong hole in her face even more appealing" (7).

This "third extraordinarily afflicted person" Rose meets within an hour of arriving in New York not only "transform[s] the difficulties of the first

     THE INVADING BODY

two meetings" (7) but also provides a model that will shape the way she is to conceive of her own illness in the future. Edna offers Rose "a home away from home" (10) that sustains her when other friends and family are too absorbed by "the crisis of their own mortality brought on by my [Rose's] illness" (104) to help. In her "quiet and undramatic" (8) way, Edna manages to lead what Rose will later call "a normally unhappy life" with the disease—unburdened by "the council of despair" of alternative healing that links survival with one's ability to "dissolve the difficulty of living, of love, of self and other, [and] of the other in the self" (105).

Her respect for Edna's approach to illness is augmented when, years later, she finds out that Edna's whole life has been an embodied defiance of the boundaries that separate the normal from the pathological. "What Edna," she says

> did not tell me then, did not tell me until several years later, after her ninety-sixth birthday, when Jim was long dead and my own circumstances had radically changed, was that she had first been diagnosed as having cancer when she was sixteen years old—in 1913. She graduated from Barnard College in 1917. How can that be—that someone with cancer since she was sixteen exudes well-being at ninety-six? Could it be because she has lived sceptically? Sceptical equally of science and of faith, of politics and of love? She has certainly not lived a perfected life. She has not been *exceptional*. She has not loved herself or others unconditionally. She has been able to go on getting it all more or less wrong, more or less all the time, all the nine and a half decades of the present century plus three years of the century before (9).

In itself "not . . . exceptional," Edna's life with cancer strikes the narrator as "an annunciation, a message" (9) at that crucial point in her life when her "own circumstances [have] radically changed." Although we learn of it much later in the narrative, the "radically changed" circumstances she speaks of consist of finding out that she, too, has cancer. Her awed reaction to Edna's life story, and the particular interpretation that she offers of it, stem from her own skeptical brush with the medical and "New Age" or alternative discourses that surround and constitute the dominant cultural conceptions of terminal illness and, consequently, also modify the telling of her illness in the narrative present tense.

"Suppose that I were now to reveal that I have AIDS, full-blown AIDS, and have been ill during most of the course of what I have related" (76), says Rose at the exact middle of the narrative. "I would lose you. I would lose you to knowledge, to fear and to metaphor. Such a revelation would result in the sacrifice of the alchemy of my art, of artistic 'control' over the setting as well as the content of your imagination. A double sacrifice of my elocution: to the unspeakable (death) and to the overspoken (AIDS)" (76–77). Unlike the themes she has touched on so far—which include forms of self-exposure and loss as painful and intimate as the loss of parents, lovers, friends, and even a whole people (in her discussion of the Holocaust)—talking about the loss of her own health apparently introduces an element of actuality that threatens to collapse, even retrospectively, the very contract she erected with her reader. However carefully she may design the moment of telling about her illness, the act of telling entails a sacrifice of her authorial control—"I would lose you"—which in turn undermines speech ("my elocution") itself. Thus, the twin risks of verbal incontinence and dissociation from language, which were previously connected with the experience of illness, have not been eliminated but rather displaced to the level of the telling. Both in terms of the reader's suspended disbelief in the artistic "alchemy," or fictitiousness of the book, and in terms of "the autobiographical pact" à la Philippe Lejeune, in which the reader is invited to test the authenticity of the identity between author, narrator, and protagonist (14), telling of one's terminal illness is perceived as dangerously self-destructive. Speaking about illness entails the replacement of authorial control with "the overspoken" and "the unspeakable," and not simply because it triggers the reader's projection of cultural "knowledge," "fear," and "metaphor" onto the text. It is disruptive, too, of the game of disclosure and equivocation the narrator has established through conscientiously leaving sufficient gaps in the telling to make the act of reading reciprocally engaging as the reader proceeds to fill in the gaps. In this sense, disclosing the fact of one's terminal illness literally threatens to stop the reading.

So far, the narrator says, "we have kept the terms of our contract: you [the reader] have given me free rein, and I have honoured my share of the obligation by not using up that freedom, by leaving large tracks of compacted equivocation at every twist in the telling" (77). But once terminal illness is introduced, it works to "deliberately spoil this narration by reduced equivocation" (77). The reductive force of telling about her illness is what the narrator would struggle with in an attempt to reassert her agency as a teller who contains the illness rather than being contained by it. In the face of both hers and the readers' acknowledgment of material fatality, her project is to celebrate life by reinstating the game of equivocation with her readers. As she immediately proceeds to say, her motivation for writing about her illness is no different from her motivation for writing at large: "I must continue to write for the same reason I am always compelled to write, in sickness and in health: for, otherwise, I die deadly, but this way, by this work, I may die forward into the intensified agon of living" (77). The motivation for writing remains the same, but in contrast with the actual course of terminal illness, writing is a way of defying closure, of defeating "deadly" death by pursuing the self-empowering game with the reader.

Accordingly, as we soon find out, her admission to having AIDS is a verbal hoax that sustains her narrative control—as does her decision to highlight the artificiality of the disclosure by placing it at the exact middle of the narrative. Moreover, even her subsequent confession to the autobiographical "truth" of having an advanced-stage cancer is couched in the conditional voice and warns against any assumption of categorical knowledge:

If I were now to explain that, in my early forties, I have cancer, say, advanced ovarian cancer, which has failed to respond to chemotherapies, and is spread throughout the peritoneum, the serous membrane lining the cavity of the abdomen, and in the pleura, the serous lining of the lungs, you would respond according to the exigencies of taxonomy, symbol, and terror, according to ignorance rather than knowledge, although there is, in fact and in spirit, no relevant knowledge. For you "cancer" means, on the one hand, a lump, a species of discrete matter with multiplying properties, [and] on the other hand, a judgement, a species of ineluctable condemnation. (78)

Ignorance prevails and no knowledge is relevant, since to respond knowledgeably to illness would require the experiential, idiosyncratic access that remains beyond the reach of anyone but the sick individual in the present tense. The "scientific" terminology that describes Rose's cancer proves no more adequate as a representation of her experience of terminal illness than do the popular "materialist" or "spiritualist" conceptions of cancer assumed by the lay reader. No wonder the narrator insists on the totally arbitrary sense of the code word *cancer*: "To the bearer of this news, the term 'cancer' means nothing: it has no meaning. It merges without remainder into the horizon within which the difficulties, the joys, the banalities, of each day elapse" (78). Yet, if the constitutive and self-referential systems of medical practice and cultural myths lag inevitably—"in fact and in spirit"—not only with the experience of having cancer but also with the ability to relate *it* and to relate *to* it, how can we hope to read Rose's *Reckoning,* even with the kind of animated, skeptical attitude she seems to endorse?

For one thing, like Edna, like Rose herself, we need to lose language in order to regain it. We have to unlearn what we know of "the 'cancer personality,' described by the junk literature of cancer" (85), since the pop spirituality of "the literature of alternative healing" betrays "poor psychology, worse theology and no notion of justice at all" (104). And we must, likewise, resist the authority of conventional medicine, whose reductive professional perspective classifies patients either as cured or as good as dead. "Surgeons," says Rose, "are not qualified for the one thing with which they deal: life. For they do not understand, as part of their profession, 'death,' in the non-medical sense, nor therefore 'life' in the meaningful sense, inclusive of death. When they fail to 'cure,' according to their own lights, they deal out death: 'You won't die at eighty of boredom.' 'Since you may well die within a year of your operation, it is not worth spoiling your remaining time with more chemotherapy that will make you deaf'" (79).

THE INVADING BODY

Exploring the crisis of illness as an aspect of life, and, further, as an opportunity to "better prepare you for the earthly impossibilities" (105), is what Rose is ultimately after in writing her autobiography. As its subtitle (*A Reckoning with Life*) suggests, she wishes to embrace "Life" in the strongest sense. Writing, for her, is an ethical force that aspires to goad the reader into seeing "the impasses, the limitations and cruelties, equally, of alternative healing and of conventional medicine" (77). More ambitiously, as she says, "I would insinuate *démarches* of healing that have not been imagined in either canon" (77). Writing, then, generates resistance, invention, the courageous loss and regaining of meaning—actions of empowerment that are nonetheless steeped in the self-consciousness of failure: "I would oppose to the iatrogenic materiality of medicine and to the screwtape overdose of spirituality of alternative healing, *love's work* [the title of her narrative], the work I have been charting, accomplishing, but, above all and necessarily, failing in, all along the way" (78).

Such a vacillation between a sense of power and of powerlessness maps the difficulty of relating to, and containing, the transformed, sick body. In *Love's Work*, the challenge of the changed body to one's sense of control is conveyed in a microcosm through Rose's attempt to account for her colostomy. This supposedly temporary procedure was part of the first operation to remove her ovarian tumor along with organs infected with metastases. The hope was that if all went well, the colostomy would then be reversed after the successful application of chemotherapy. That hope was frustrated, but in choosing to write about it, Rose endeavors to contain through language that which medical intervention has rendered incontinent. By articulating the condition of physical incontinence, she aspires at once to come to terms with "the re-siting of bodily function" and to extricate her private experience from the encroaching public discourses of distaste, the medical textbook, and altogether "too much interest" (94). The discussion of colostomy is significant since it is an example of how Rose writes about her illness synecdochically: through the colostomy discussion, she shows readers how she tries to grapple with a much more dire physical change and the way it affects one's thinking, one's rhetoric, and thus, even one's identity. Yet, while she finds that describing how a colostomy looks "is comparatively easy to put into prose because it is likely to be utterly unfamiliar," she seems unable to answer the key question of "[h]ow to inscribe my relation to its [the colostomy's] operation" (94). The harder she tries to articulate her relation to the changed body, the farther she seems to get from an account of her condition in the present tense.

Once she dismisses "the overworked cliché of a changed body image," which, as she says, "relates to motor and imaginary self-representation, and not to the re-siting of bodily function" (94), she can verbalize her relation to her present condition only by contrasting it with the "normal" past: "What having a colostomy makes you realise is that normally you bear hardly any relation to your excrement . . . It is the sphincter muscle which affords the self-relation of retention and release. To exchange this discretion for an anterior cloaca and incontinence . . . how easy it is to borrow the prepared associations" (95). It is as if one's body, arguably the most familiar and intimate aspect of identity, remains constantly out of reach, estranged from the self either by the instinctive, preverbal "self-relation of retention and release" or by the resort to "prepared associations" (95). Still, the dysfunctional body is what provokes the realization of the acute discrepancy between present and past, sickness and health. In other words, one's experience of the changed body in illness triggers knowledge of the body as it existed before that change. But at the same time, the experience of illness functions as the source for the very desire to relate to the sick body in the narrative present tense.

The desire to respond to her physical experience by clearing a discursive space for what she terms "the uncharted" governs Rose's telling of her colostomy. It is coupled, however, with her fear of failing to maintain a balance between excessive speech and unwelcoming reserve. This is not just a question of saying too much or too little but also, crucially, of how the telling might be (mis)read. "I want to talk about shit—the hourly transfiguration of our lovely eating of the sun. I need to remove the discourse of shit from transgression, sexual fetishism, from too much interest, but, equally, from coyness, distaste and the medical textbook. My interest is in the uncharted; my difficulty that I will inevitably enlist, by connotation and implication, the power and grace of the symbol. I need to invent colostomy ethnography" (94). Clearly, Rose's interest in "the

THE INVADING BODY

uncharted" here is larger than the specific subject at hand. Her focus on the "need to invent colostomy ethnography" retrieves the desire to construct an inverted ratio between one's loss of control over the body and the regaining of a verbal hold over the experience of such loss. However, in the attempt to "describe a new bodily function, not to redescribe the old" (95), she is inevitably caught in the available cultural network that links the dysfunctional body with the obscene. Once again, the twin risks of giving in either to the unspeakable ("coyness, distaste") or to the overspoken ("too much interest"), which were previously shown as threatening one's authorship of the telling of one's illness, cause her to engage in a conscious struggle against the compelling power of silence, on one hand, and of "prepared associations" (95), on the other.

A major device Rose employs to counter the force of the unspeakable and the overspoken is disclosed in her particular use of analogy. The discussion of her colostomy is preceded by a seemingly unrelated account of the Holocaust scholar Robert Jan van Pelt, whose study of Auschwitz architectural plans led him "to emphasize the contingent nature of many features of the so-called 'Holocaust,' which our use of holistic periphrasis tends to represent as predetermined and overly rational" (92). Yet, Rose remarks, at the very moment van Pelt raises the contingency of items such as the infamous barbed wire at the perimeter of the camp and the inadequate sanitation in the men's and women's barracks at Birkenau, which "resulted in much *unplanned* death," he is caught,

> inadvertently but predictably . . . in the tightening coils of Holocaust ethnography. . . . Caught, above all, concerning the practicalities of excrement, or, as he tersely puts it, concerning the subject of shit. People, he reports, are relatively inured to discussions of the design of gas chambers and inefficiency in the operation of the four crematoria. Yet . . . when he raises issues relating to the mismanagement of sanitation at the camps, he is met with reluctance, embarrassment and loss of attention (92).

Immediately following this passage, and without any other comment concerning the Holocaust, Rose launches the telling of her colostomy.

Thus juxtaposed, her discussion of colostomy is colored by the inevitable parallels with van Pelt's argumentation. Like van Pelt, she focuses on the unheroic, possibly humiliating, and clearly unplanned aspect of a major event—her colostomy was contingent on the surgery she underwent to remove the tumor. And she, too, confronts the problematic of "the subject of shit": on the one hand, the audience's reluctant response, embarrassment, and loss of attention; on the other hand, "the tightening coils" (92) of superfluous meaning—"transgression, sexual fetishism" and "too much interest" (94).

This is not to say that the use of analogy here establishes a direct relationship between Holocaust and cancer ethnography, or between death in the camps and medical surgery. To suggest that would be not only ludicrous but obstructive to the game of disclosure and equivocation that Rose wishes to enact with her readers. Rose herself works against an overt analogy when she lays claim to "the uncharted." "Nowhere in the endless romance of world literature," she declares, "have I come across an account of living with a colostomy" (93). If van Pelt's research is complicated by the already existing "coils of Holocaust ethnography," Rose's problem is "to invent colostomy ethnography" in the first place, although she is conscious of failing to do so in the sense that her idiosyncratic physical experience will inevitably be tainted by the "always already" surrounding discourses. Nonetheless, the analogy she alternately evokes and evades opens a space for her to engage the reader in a search for meaning, and where, moreover, the reader's identification and sympathy for her undertaking become a feasible possibility. "The uncharted," in this sense, is that extratextual space of cognitive and emotive meaning, which is yet to be met by the reader.

This opening up of her narrative to readerly participation seems at first sight to contrast with Rose's previously noted fascination with anticipating and controlling her audience's response. But that is because her narrative shifts between two distinct and, at times, exclusive meanings of *control:* control in terms of managing others and determining their response and control in the sense of taking in "an initially unwelcome event," "some damage or trauma," and making it "one's own inner occupation" (98). The collapse of normal bodily functions engenders an

THE INVADING BODY

opportunity for learning control in the second sense and considerably reduces the need to attain control in the first sense. Thus, when Rose emerges from anesthesia after her second operation and waits to hear from her doctors about the perceived effects of the chemotherapy, she is anxious to have "control over the broadcasting of any ambiguities" (98). However, as the three specialists who treat her persist in giving conflicting judgments of her condition, and no amount of pleading, cajoling, begging, and flattering help to reconcile their "utterly discrepant" (102) diagnoses, she realizes—notably, in the narrative present tense—that "my light lies in their discrepancy" (102). At this moment of apparent total dependence on the agency of others, the second sense of "control" affords a healing power in that it accelerates her departure from "the disintegrating authority of conventional medicine" (102), thereby enabling her to assert her agency as "a broadcaster" herself.

"Medicine and I have dismissed each other," she says. "We do not have enough command of each other's language for the exchange to be fruitful" (102). Pragmatically, this means that she decides to forgo further courses of treatment; yet her decision stems not from a sense of despair but rather from a determination to resume her life. If medical diagnosis can be viewed as both "a linguistic entity, a declaration of judgment, and a plan for action in the real world" (Treichler, "Escaping" 71)—implying a linear movement from speech act to literal action—the impasse created by Rose's conflicting diagnoses triggers in her the reverse motion: from being literally silenced and operated on, anesthetized only to wake up "screaming with physical and mental distress" (101), she moves to reclaim both her body and her discourse. "If I am mute, then so is medicine. It can no more fathom my holistic and spiritual matrix than I can master its material syntax. I must return to my life affair" (103). As her narrative attests, "mute" she evidently is not, although the "life affair" in which she wishes to reinscribe herself continues to present the risk of losing control either in the sense of having priority over others or in the more subtle sense of "taking in." The "fatal language of clinical control" (104) exercises power only in the first sense, notably by instituting and monitoring the division between the separate spheres of illness and health. By contrast, the "more elusive" sense that Rose learns to look for—"a sense," she insists, that "saves my life" (98)—is concerned with the ability to attend to one's finality.

"It is power to be able *to attend,* powerful or powerless" (135), she says in the chapter that ends her autobiography. In this chapter she offers a critique of the "authority of relativism" in postmodern philosophy, which apparently has no immediate bearing on the subject of illness. Nonetheless, the chapter enacts the very terms under which the discussion of illness was conceived. Returning, finally, to doing philosophy—to her life's work—Rose dramatizes her perception of illness as a life affair, an ongoing tending to "the agon of living." The repeated term *agon,* which is used interchangeably in the text to indicate both writing and "Life," deserves further clarification, since it not only renders Rose's existential stance throughout the narrative but distinguishes this stance from the organizing paradigms—that of the battle and of the athletic ideal—commonly found in illness narratives. As a philosopher who pays scrupulous attention to words, Rose is evidently aware of the etymological derivation of the term *agon* that encompasses the notions of both "assembly" and "contest" (Nagy 57). She notes, for example, that the Greek *agora* means "the market-place, the place of assembly" (132), and specifically adds that "it implies public, articulate space, space full of interconnections" (132). Her agon of living, then, is not a battlefield or an enclosed arena in which her illness is to be fought out, but, rather, a relational space that requires the rhetorical skills of a classical orator combined with a modern, modest readiness to embrace "the risk of relation: that mix of exposure and reserve, of revelation and reticence" (105) that applies equally to self-writing and to love. Crucially unlike the paradigms of a battle or an athletic contest, her notion of agon does not afford the consoling, wish-fulfilling element of a future terminus, of an end to the game, "when . . . the player or patient will simply return to an ordinary life in 'the real world'" (Hawkins 77). The real world, for Rose, is just this self-reflexive engagement in an ongoing contest among competing discourses, which subsumes and surpasses the prevailing cultural constructs. Indeed, the saving power of her autobiography lies in her ability to admit the self-imposed vulnerability and risks entailed in exposing one's terminal illness and, at the same time,

THE INVADING BODY

to recast the telling of her illness in terms that cross the boundaries of sickness and health.

For the reader, the reality effect of the narrative is established at those moments when the telling itself collapses, when the narrator's game of equivocation, however earnest, is replaced by her fear of reduction. It is here that the narrating self overlaps with the identity of Rose the author. It is here, moreover, that the reader is directed to the experiential basis of her illness narrative. Viewed in this light, Rose's autobiography reacts against the insulating tendency of the genre to preserve the writers' and the readers' sense of equanimity by employing a predictable paradigm or narrative frame. As a consequence, her discourse falls short of the sub-genre's conscious intention to help others who are ill or who witness the illness of relatives and friends. Her narrative's thematic complexity and formal innovations—many of which were left out of this discussion for lack of space[3]—may be too far removed from the pragmatic, or the immediately political concerns of the ill. Even her tone—sophisticated, urbane, often bemused—is unlikely to find an easy path to the hearts of bereaved relatives and friends. Yet, if Rose's implied readers are taxed by the need to unlearn, or at least to revise, their conventional view of illness, this may well be a blessing in disguise. By opening up the genre to a diversity of audiences, and by challenging its formal tendency to "perpetuate pre-modernist conventions" (Couser, *Recovering* 293), *Love's Work* not only serves to integrate the representation of the experience of illness in the broad realm of contemporary literature,[4] but also, more subtly, it works against the cultural processes that marginalize and infantilize the ill themselves.

2

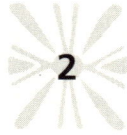

FIRST YOU HURT

THIS DISCUSSION OF ILLNESS NARRATIVES WOULD NOT BE COM-
plete without an acknowledgment of the groundbreaking contribution of
feminist theory to the current understanding of embodiment in social
and humanistic studies as a historically and culturally constructed process of materialization. Feminist philosophers such as Iris Young, Judith
Butler, Elizabeth Grosz, Susan Bordo, and Luce Irigaray have analyzed
the pretensions and illusions of western ideals of epistemological objectivity and phenomenological neutrality and uncovered the residual force
of Cartesian dualism in specific social contexts and practices that produce, rather than reflect, gendered marks of embodiment.[1] Theirs, and
many others',[2] systematic critiques of the binary constructions of mind/
body, reason/nature, man/woman, outside/inside dualities have resulted
in stressing, in Elizabeth Grosz's words, "that the generic category, '*the
body*' is a masculinist illusion" ("Psychoanalysis and the Body" 270). In
uncovering the universalization of a masculinist body in western philosophical tradition, furthermore, feminist theory has underscored the
way "[c]onditions of embodiment are organized by systemic patterns of
domination and sub-ordination, making it impossible to grasp individual
body practices, body regimes and discourses about the body without taking power into account" (Davis, "Embody-ing" 14). Thus reconceived as

a "socio-cultural artifact" that is produced and developed through "various regimes of discipline and training" (Grosz, "Bodies-Cities" 103, 104), the body and its boundaries have been extricated from their traditional identification with biological immanence, inert nature, and the generic female. *Embodiment* has largely replaced *the body* as a key term that encompasses the temporal, relational, acquired, and potentially plural aspects of the corporeal self.[3]

Feminist political practice, moreover, paved the way for consciousness-raising activities and political writing organized and produced by disabled and sick people.[4] As Susan Bordo has pointed out, the prevailing argument that ideas are created by social beings who belong to hierarchized social groups can be traced to the emancipatory liberation movements of the 1960s and 1970s.[5] Inspired by the transformative political agency of the 1960s liberation movements, cultural critics and disabled people have recognized ableism and ageism as oppressive social constructs that cut across individual lives in ways similar to class-, race-, and sex-based structures of cultural oppression.[6] Once we accept that "[m]odern philosophy and science established unifying, controlling reason in opposition to and mastery over the body, and then identified some [social] groups with reason and others with the body" (Young, *Justice* 124), we can begin to see that, as a social group, sick and disabled people are especially vulnerable to forms of cultural imperialism.[7]

Clearly associated not only with the devalued category of the body but also with the subcategory of the ailing body, sick and disabled people are marked as Others. As Iris Marion Young emphasizes throughout her *Justice and the Politics of Difference,* in a culture consciously committed to the liberal imperative of equality and respect for all social groups, much of the aversive behavior directed toward oppressed groups occurs either unconsciously or at a level of practical consciousness embodied in various gestures of avoidance. "The liberal imperative that differences should make no difference puts a sanction of silence on those things which at the level of practical consciousness people 'know' about the significance of group differences" (134), says Young. Thus, like other oppressed groups such as women, blacks, gays, lesbians, and old people, disabled and sick people "not only suffer the humiliation of aversive, avoiding, or condescending behavior, but must usually experience that behavior in silence, unable to check their perceptions against those of others" (134).

Illness narratives are political agents for change insofar as they allow sick and disabled people to break the sanction of silence and bring their experience of cultural oppression to the level of discursive consciousness. Unlike racially and sexually oppressed groups, however, sick people have a unique vantage point on their cultural interpellation as "despised, deformed, or fearful bodies," a status Young believes all inferiorized groups occupy as a crucial element of their oppression (*Justice,* 142). This is because unlike other subalterns, such as women or people of color, people with critical illnesses often experience quite suddenly the deleterious transition from occupying the unmarked status of good health to being identified, and identifying themselves, with the marked and silenced group of the disabled. (Sometimes, indeed, they also enjoy the reverse transition and rejoin the superior group of the able-bodied). Such a peculiarly fraught experience of social mobility gives writers of illness narratives a phenomenological leverage on issues of bodily inscription. Their experiential accounts of sick bodies, in other words, can test poststructuralist and feminist formulations of the cultural source of our commitments to the morphological categorization of the body into social groups.

In an article entitled "Our Bodies, Ourselves: Why We Should Add Old Fashioned Empirical Phenomenology to the New Theories of the Body," Helen Marshall rightly observes that the poststructuralist feminist project of theorizing the body "tends to be either from a psychoanalytic perspective, or from the external approach that takes bodies as texts," making "disturbingly little reference to empirical work that comes from the tradition of phenomenology" (64). I agree with Marshall that neither the "external approach" nor "speculative writing from the psychoanalytic version of the 'internal'" relies on investigation of "how the body is experienced as a way of getting a better theoretical hold on the concept" (Marshall 64). While most feminists researching the body today would agree with Maurice Merleau-Ponty that "[t]he body is our general medium for having a world" (*Phenomenology* 146, qtd. in Moi 63), their focus on how bodies are psychically and culturally produced distances them from the

THE INVADING BODY

concrete lived experiences of individuals in the social world, that is, from "attending to individuals' actual material bodies or their everyday interactions with their bodies and through their bodies with the world around them" (Davis, "Embody-ing" 15). However, the problem is not merely, as Davis points out, that embodiment theories fail to "tackle the relationship between the symbolic and the material, between representations of the body and embodiment as experience" ("Embody-ing" 15). Even more pressing is the implicit denial or effacement of the possible significance of such relationships since bodies are conceived to be mere products or effects of an always already regulating discursivity.[8] From this perspective it is no wonder that endeavors to explore the subversive symbolic possibilities of the body are privileged over empirical phenomenological accounts of lived experience.[9]

The significance of illness narratives, however, is in the various ways they demonstrate that if embodiment theories are not anchored in the immediacies of everyday life, research on the body is virtually bound to be trapped into idealizing the body as an abstraction. In focusing on bodies as objects of social knowledge, as cultural constructs that are "plastic, malleable and amenable to social re-inscription" (Grosz "Psychoanalysis and the Body" 270), "external" theories of embodiment often lead to a conceptual slippage that results in altogether negating the body as a medium for knowledge and, particularly, as a source of certain kinds of knowledge. Illness narratives provide a corrective to this by insisting on the difference between thinking about and living the experience of individual bodies. In reminding their audience that life-threatening illness is not a metaphor, in their conscious desire "to demetaphorize . . . [a] life journey, which includes death" (Middlebrook 206), writers of illness narratives alert us to questions of affectivity and pragmatics, rather than of epistemology, in respect to the lived body. This is surely not to say that cultural constructs become irrelevant in these texts. Certainly, illness narratives also make clear that while sick people share a specific group history and identity, they also hold other memberships to other culturally inferiorized groups. As Janet Price and Margrit Shildrick have remarked, "[g]iven that all women are positioned in relation to and measured against an inaccessible body ideal, in part determined by a universalised male body, the experience of female disablement as such may be seen as the further marginalisation of the already marginal" (433). That "[i]n relation to the 'whole' body of phenomenology, women with disabilities may be seen as doubly dis-abled" (Price and Shildrick 435) is a particular facet of Grosz's general assertion that when we speak of bodily inscription we must bear in mind that "[t]here is no 'natural' norm; there are only cultural forms of body, which do or do not conform to social norms" (*VB* 143). Yet how do these epistemological observations help us to understand the pragmatics of embodied practices and lived experience in concrete situations? And how may women's autobiographical accounts of bodily limitation, such as memoirs, journals, and letters, enter the discussion of corporeal subjectivity and test the current trend in feminist theory to discard empirical phenomenology in the name of an antihumanism that conceives of the body first and foremost as a social and discursive product?

My reading of dozens of women's accounts of their experience of illness and medical treatment has made me realize that these women's sense of extreme vulnerability, alienation, and marginalization in illness vigorously challenges the poststructuralist-feminist injunction to reject the body as a source of knowledge and to identify embodied practices with (conformist or subversive) constitutive performance. Ironically, some women find contemporary feminist theory itself to be alienating and alienated, unable to account for their experiences in a sick body. For Susan Wendell, for example, the experience of illness clashes with the tendency she identifies in feminist theory to conceive of the body as "limited only by the imagination," a tendency that "ignores bodily experience altogether" (325). Wendell testifies that

> When I became ill, I felt taken over and betrayed by a profound bodily vulnerability. I was forced by my body to reconceptualize my relationship to it. This experience was not the result of any change of cultural "reading" of the body or of technological incursions into the body. . . . Of course, my illness occurred in a social and cultural context, which profoundly affected my experience of it, but a major aspect of my experience was precisely that of being forced to acknowledge and learn

to live with *bodily,* not cultural, limitation. In its radical movement away from the view that every facet of women's lives is determined by biology, feminist theory is in danger of idealizing "the body" and erasing much of the reality of lived bodies. (325)

To affirm, as Wendell does, the profound role of bodily limitations in constituting lived experience does not mean, as some feminists might fear, that biological facts form the scientific (essentialist) ground from which subjectivity is derived and by which it is determined. It means, rather, that our continual encounter with the way the body is felt, which becomes exceptionally persistent in illness, highlights the relationship of contingency and contiguity between subjectivity and biological processes.[10]

The following discussion of specific autobiographical accounts of the experience of living with breast cancer will show that the contingent and contiguous relationship between subjectivity and bodily disintegration does not entail unified, "generic," or monistic experience. Rather, this relationship defines the experiencing subject, who, placed in concrete circumstances, seeks her particular way of being with illness and learns to develop, as best she can, the strategies of self-defense that best suit her situation. I have chosen to concentrate in this chapter on breast-cancer journals partly because of the normative cultural construction of breasts in Western patriarchy as the supreme visual mark of femininity. In the case of breast cancer, the (initial) location of disease in the breast and the physical and mental effects of the commonly prescribed procedures of mastectomy, radiation, and chemotherapy emphasize the highly complex reality of interrelatedness between organic processes, bodily practices, and the various cultural and institutional constructions of illness, health, sexual specificity, and self-identity. Breast-cancer journals thus present a synthetic view of lived experience that advances feminist thinking beyond the essence/construction debate. By underlining the contingent relationship between bodies and subjectivities in specific, and changing, situations, breast-cancer journals corroborate Merleau-Ponty's concept of lived experience, which, in Grosz's words, "is not outside social, political, historical, and cultural forces" and yet should be addressed by theory not "as something to be explained away as simply untrustworthy or 'ideological' but as something to be explained" (*VB* 95). My reading of these narratives, therefore, does not resort to naive formulations of mimesis and authorial intention but treats the phenomenological, experiencing subject as constituted at once by discursive practices and physiological conditions.

The first part of this discussion juxtaposes conflicting autobiographical accounts of breast amputation and breast reconstruction as narrated in Audre Lorde's *The Cancer Journals* and Musa Mayer's *Examining Myself: One Woman's Story of Breast Cancer Treatment and Recovery*. My reading is framed by insights gleaned from the feminist debate over the empowering or injurious effects of the practice of cosmetic surgery on women's politics and individual sense of agency. I argue, however, that unless we inquire into women's lived experiences of mastectomy and breast implantation, such as are attended to in breast-cancer memoirs, the controversy will remain abstract and politically ineffectual. The problem of voicing lived experience in language will dominate the second part of the chapter, which addresses the paradoxical need of women with advanced, metastatic cancer to demetaphorize their experience of illness and yet to verbalize the sick body in terms of the physiological, emotional, existential, and interpersonal effects of living with a life-threatening disease. My reading of breast-cancer journals by Barbara Rosenblum, Christina Middlebrook, Treya Killam Wilber, and others considers recent feminist explorations of the central role played by body image as a mediating concept between organic processes and subjectivity, and these explorations' relevance to individual endeavors of trying to make sense of fatal illness. This is not to say that the conflicts triggered by bodily experience are finally resolved or reconciled by "better" theoretical formulations. The usefulness of reading illness narratives lies in their power to show that, while we cannot ignore the varied meanings of embodied states, bodies are messy rather than theoretically neat. Consequently, it is futile to approach these narratives in terms of a one-to-one application of theory to illustrative texts. A more promising, though much more modest, approach is to adhere to personal accounts of illness on their own terms. In privileging experiential accounts of bodily limitation, this section embraces Wendell's call to "recognize that awareness of the body is often awareness of pain, discomfort, or physical difficulty," and that "[s]ince people with disabilities collectively have a great deal of knowledge about these aspects of bodily experience, they should be major contributors to our cultural understanding of the body" (326).

MASTECTOMY AND ITS AFTERMATH

Within mainstream constructionist feminism, the debate over cosmetic surgery is conducted between, on the one hand, the majority of feminist cultural critics, who view cosmetic surgery as self-inflicting subordination to the patriarchal beauty system, and, on the other, a minority of critics who argue against seeing women as victims or gulls of ideological oppression. Thus, Susie Orbach, Kathryn Morgan, Susan Brownmiller, and Susan Bordo, while placing different emphases on the practical and ideological aspects of Western culture's discourses of femininity, agree that since women are taught from an early age to view their bodies as commodities, their ability to resist the system of beauty norms, let alone make an informed and genuine choice in respect to cosmetic surgery, is limited.[11] Kathy Davis and Dorothy Smith, on the other hand, grant women an active role in remedying their dissatisfaction with their bodies.[12] Davis in particular approaches cosmetic surgery as a legitimate means of rectifying the felt gap between cultural pressures on how women should look and women's sense of bodily deficiency. Altering the body through surgery, that is, is perceived by Davis as an extension of more traditional skills of "doing femininity."[13] Although she admits that she remains "critical of the practice of cosmetic surgery and the discourse of feminine inferiority which it sustains," Davis regards individual women who undergo cosmetic surgery as active and knowledgeable agents capable of seeing through patriarchal conditions of oppression even as they comply with them. In the course of her interviews with women before and after surgery, she "learned of their despair, not because their bodies were not beautiful, but because they were not ordinary—'just like everyone else'" ("Cosmetic Surgery" 455). She concludes that, for these women, cosmetic surgery offers "a way to reinstate a damaged sense of self and become who they really are or should have been" (*Reshaping* 169).

Women's experiential accounts of mastectomy invariably disclose their injured self-image and feelings of loss, envy, and nostalgia for their old, "ordinary" selves. According to Davis's view of cosmetic surgery, and against mainstream feminism that closes the debate by marking the politically correct line, these women are excellent candidates for the benefits offered by surgical breast reconstruction. (Many women today are in fact encouraged by their plastic surgeons to have a tissue expander inserted in preparation for the artificial breast implant while they are still anaesthetized, immediately following their mastectomy.) My reading about women's experiences of mastectomy and breast reconstruction, however, leads me to think that the disparity between these women's "public persona"—the appearance of normalcy defined by elevated standards of femininity—and "the secret wounds" (Mayer 129) of their embodied selves is far from resolved by the act of wearing a prosthesis or undergoing breast reconstruction. The problem with Davis's approach to cosmetic surgery is that her sequential connection between surgically altered appearance, how women are viewed by others, and women's attainment of a sense of "who they really are or should have been" confuses cultural representations of women's bodies with the way women experience their changed bodies over time. Granted, our body image is also the result of shared sociocultural conceptions of bodies (Grosz, *VB* 84), but neither body images nor bodily experiences are simply equivalent to culturally prescribed bodily styles. I believe that since mastectomy and breast reconstruction following a diagnosis of cancer involve women's heightened awareness of mortality and of bodily vulnerability, these women's experiential accounts can teach us more about the complexity of their lived relationship with their bodies than can the cases of "pure" cosmetic surgery that Davis has examined. Experiential accounts of mastectomy, moreover, highlight the contiguous relationship between bodies and subjectivity that occurs also in "normal" healthy life. As Iris Marion Young has argued in "Breasted Experience: The Look and the Feeling," even "normal" breasted experience is an ambivalent reality, conditioned by the objectifying gaze of the dominant male subject and yet inseparable from the way women experience their breasts in terms of sensitivity, touch, and bodily movement (192–93).[14]

To a large extent, the more focused feminist controversy over breast reconstruction does not take into account that breast implantation is not only about a woman's initial decision to undergo reconstructive surgery but also involves various medical interventions and emotionally and physically unpredictable responses over a substantial period of time—sometimes extending over two years—until the process of implantation is completed. Similarly, neither those who oppose reconstructive surgery nor those who uphold women's ability to arrive at an informed decision about it inquire into these women's lived experience of surgery and their relationship to their mastectomy and artificial breast after medical intervention has been concluded. On each side of the debate, speakers center their arguments on the degree of agency individual women may have when they attempt to make an informed decision about breast implantation surgery: they analyze the phallocentric beauty ideals that, cynically enforced by the medical system, annul women's choice and voluntary consent, or point to the problematic paternalistic ethics of trying to dictate to women the politically correct line.

For those who wish to affirm women's agency and choice, the pain and health risks that reconstructive surgery entails are effaced by the assumption that the benefits of breast implantation surgery are largely subjective and constituted by whether the woman herself thinks that surgery serves her interests. In other words, they conceive of women's individual interests and actions as ethically prior to the collective interests of women. Thus, while Lisa S. Parker concedes that "[a] woman's choice of implantation will, of course, help construct a culture in which women's (re)constructions of their bodies, at risk to their health, are acceptable responses to other cultural constructions," she nonetheless asserts that "the alternative of not respecting women's choice to have breast implants as voluntary, competent decisions is even more unacceptable": "To refuse to accept women's consent to breast implant surgery as valid, one would have to either deny their agency or their competence as decision makers" (266).

Parker's position exemplifies a typical impasse in certain strands of constructionist feminism, one reached also by Davis and Smith. On the one hand, she perceives social reality in terms of an intricate network of power relations that shape and affect individual compliance with social norms, while on the other hand, she cannot entirely give up the liberal (and feminist) emancipatory ideal of individual choice and agency. Yet, attending to women's narratives of living with breast cancer, rather than to what is deemed theoretically "unacceptable," reveals that "informed decision" in respect to breast implantation is a contradiction in terms. Not only can women not arrive at genuine judgments about their reconstructive surgery until after it has taken place, but even after the painstakingly long and physically and emotionally challenging process of inflation, implantation, mastopexy (reconstructive surgery in the healthy breast for better symmetry), nipple reconstruction, and tattooing is finally completed, the reality of living with the consequences of breast reconstruction is often fettered by uncertainty and self-doubt.

Women who write about their experiences of illness and treatment choices often testify that they have learned to approach the whole notion of choice as a dubious construct. They acknowledge, moreover, that truths about how one would want to be treated are opaque to both "normal," healthy individuals and the sick person herself. As Treya Killam Wilber admits in her breast-cancer memoir, "I have learned that I can never know in advance what choice I would make when in someone else's place," and, furthermore, "I didn't choose what *I* thought I would have chosen either" (253). Women's accounts of their concrete experiences of mastectomy and other treatment choices are nonetheless useful for readers who are forced to make similar decisions and for scholars engaged in embodiment theories and feminist politics of transformation. Their testimonies of the felt effects of illness and treatment provide extreme test cases of embodied experience that may confirm or problematize abstract conceptions of "normative" corporeal subjectivity at large. In addition, the narrators in these texts pose explicit demands for social change that would widen the range of treatment choices they can have and make the available cultural constructions of normative femininity fit better with their altered embodied identity.

More than twenty years ago, Audre Lorde stated in a frequently cited sentence that "[w]hen I mourn my right breast, it is not the appearance of it I mourn, but the feeling and the fact" (64–65). Lorde's *The Cancer Journals,* from which this sentence is quoted, is a personal and political denouncement of our culture's privileging of normative feminine appearance and its concomitant silencing of the physical and psychic experiential reality of breast amputation, which is further complicated by the consciousness of death. "Any woman who has had a breast removed because of cancer knows she does not feel the same" (57), she says. Such an experiential knowledge is inconsistent with the "emphasis upon the cosmetic after surgery [which] reinforces this society's stereotype of women that we are only what we look, so this is the only aspect of our existence we need to address" (57). Lorde argues, further, that the "cosmetic sham" of prosthesis and the far more dangerous procedure of breast implantation are ways of keeping women with breast cancer invisible, silent, and separate from one another. Her own diagnosis of cancer, and particularly her mastectomy and postmastectomy experiences, ground her demand for social and political change in the lived consequences of embodied difference:

Prosthesis offers the empty comfort of "Nobody will know the difference." But it is that very difference which I wish to affirm, because I have lived it, and survived it, and wish to share that strength with other women. . . . By accepting the mask of prosthesis, one-breasted women proclaim ourselves as insufficients dependent upon pretense. We reinforce our own isolation and invisibility from each other, as well as the false complacency of a society which would rather not face the results of its own insanities. In addition, we withhold that visibility and support from one another which is such an aid to perspective and self-acceptance. Surrounded by other women day by day, all of whom appear to have two breasts, it is very difficult sometimes to remember that I AM NOT ALONE. (61)

In underlining her lived experience of mastectomy and its aftermath as inextricable from the development of her oppositional consciousness, Lorde is distinguished from the more recent bulk of constructionist feminist critics who examine women's bodily practices as signifiers of culturally constructed difference from an "external," disembodied perspective. It is through her own experience of embodied difference that she writes of the need for a political change that would make social practices fit better with women's postmastectomy experiential reality.

Surprisingly, Lorde's well-known affirmation of experiential difference and her call on one-breasted women to reclaim their bodies have had little impact on current feminist critiques of medical practices and cultural discourses, the same practices and discourses that are at work in constituting women's postmastectomy lives. Even as the incidence of breast cancer continues to rise in overwhelming numbers while the cure rate hardly changes at all (Steingraber 93–94),[15] and as reports of potentially serious health hazards concerning breast implants continue to surface in the media, feminist academics in general leave breast-cancer issues to grassroots groups of activists, most of whom are sick with breast cancer themselves. Calls to women, such as Sandra Bartky's in *Femininity and Domination,* to create a model of feminine beauty that celebrates diversity have become rare. As Toril Moi observes in *What Is a Woman?* even the word *woman* is banned from feminist discourse because of the prevalent belief in feminist theory today that "any use of the word 'woman' . . . must entail a philosophical commitment to metaphysics and essentialism" (7).

In this critical climate, the feminist debate over breast implantation veers away from the question of which alternative models of breastlessness may be acceptable to postmastectomy women. The result of this oversight is an unwanted increase in the authority and influence of surgeons, and in their self-interested participation in the normative beauty system. As Parker correctly recognizes, "a surgeon's risk-tolerant values, employed in interpreting data and disclosing risks, might poorly protect her patient's welfare and ability to make informed decisions" (61). Even after the FDA issued a requirement, in 1990, for "pre-market approval" of silicone gel implants and the polyurethane foam that coats "Même" and "Replicon" implants and may break down in the body into TDA, a known carcinogen (Mayer 125), feminist research on the body continues to ignore the particularities of medical, political, and economic issues that directly affect women's health and lived experience.

Such concrete details of everyday experience are the hallmark of breast-cancer journals. In her 1980 book, Audre Lorde recounts the crucial days immediately following mastectomy, "this period of quasi-numbness and almost childlike susceptibility to ideas" when "many patterns and net-

THE INVADING BODY

works are started for women . . . that encourage us to deny the realities of our bodies which have just been driven home to us so graphically" (41). On the third day after her mastectomy, Lorde is visited by a representative of these stereotyping "patterns and networks"—a kindly volunteer from Reach for Recovery who encourages her to wear a prosthesis, assuring her first that "nobody'll know the difference," and then "*You'll* never know the difference" (42). Even Lorde, a self-conscious and critical observer of dominant culture and its values, was at first persuaded to try on the prosthesis: "I had thought, well perhaps they know something that I don't and maybe they're right, if I put it on maybe I'll feel entirely different" (44). Her sensation when she does is that the "awkwardly inert" object that "perched on my chest askew" had "nothing to do with any me I could possibly conceive of" (44). As she looks down at herself on removing the prosthesis, she perceives that she "looked strange and uneven and peculiar to myself, but somehow, ever so much more myself, and therefore so much more acceptable, than I looked with that thing stuck inside my clothes. For not even the most skillful prosthesis in the world could undo that reality, or feel the way my breast had felt, and either I would love my body one-breasted now, or remain forever alien to myself" (44).

The same kinds of social pressure to quickly assume normative appearance right after mastectomy continue to be exerted on women with breast cancer today. Only now, women are not merely pressed to attach "a wad of lambswool" (Lorde 42) to their breastless chest but are encouraged to undertake the far more dangerous and painful procedure of breast reconstruction. Often, too, they are encouraged by the available medical literature, and pressed by their surgeon, to make up their minds about breast reconstruction before the mastectomy operation itself, in order to spare them (and the medical system) an additional operation. Thus, they are denied the privilege and the right of coming to terms with their post-mastectomy bodies. As Musa Mayer notes in *Examining Myself*, "[o]ne of the drawbacks of immediate reconstruction is that a woman makes the choice to do it with only a partial and conceptual knowledge of the alternative, and at a time when she is under great emotional pressure. She never really knows what it would be like for her to have only a scar where her breast once was, or to wear a prosthesis" (114).

In 1993, three-and-a-half years after having an artificial breast implant inserted following a mastectomy operation, Mayer still struggles with her frustrated expectation that her reconstructed breast would give her "not only the appearance of normalcy, but normalcy itself" (114). In her breast-cancer journal, Mayer vividly narrates the various surgical procedures she had to undergo during the two years of reconstruction and reveals her ambivalent reaction to the "finished" breast, which "looked okay," but does not have much feeling: "when I touched the nipple, the only thing I felt was my hand, as if I were touching someone else" (119). Over the months of her chemotherapy, the discrepancy between the symbolic meaning she attached to her reconstructed breast "as a metaphor for my whole sense of self" and the objectifying physical sensation of "the rigid grapefruit-half on my chest . . . the strange insensate mound formed by the tissue expander" (114) gradually evolved into the realization that "I was expecting an awful lot from that pound of flesh, salt water and silicone gel" (114). "I was the same person—sort of, until you looked closely—but my inner landscape had radically changed. Never had the division between outward appearance and inner experience been more sharply defined" (114).

Mayer recalls her defensive rejection of Lorde's essay on the politics of prosthesis and reconstruction in *The Cancer Journals,* which she was given a year after her diagnosis of cancer. At the time, she says, "I didn't like being told that I had been duped into a dangerous complacency" (122). She determined to affirm her "own choices" and not to worry about "the feminist 'correctness'" of her decision to undertake an immediate breast reconstruction (123). At the end of the reconstructive process, however, she admits that surgery never granted her what she really wanted: to go back to being "as I used to be, the woman who could hike and dance and lose weight and feel the spontaneous flush of sexual desire" (121). As she traces her two-year obsession with the reconstructed breast to her irreversibly changed "inner sense of femaleness" (120), she begins to see that reconstructive surgery had become for her "the single positive visual symbol that might stave off the desexualization process that had begun years before with my hysterectomy" (120). The reality of living with her reconstructed breast belies the tantalizing promise of the

THE INVADING BODY

operation to medically resurrect not only the primary symbol of femininity but also her collapsed "sexual body image" (120), namely, her lived experience of diminishment in sexual interest and responsiveness and "the kind of confidence that flows naturally from being healthy and fit and attractive" (121).

Although she comes to enjoy touching the artificial breast—"[s]omehow, with the sensations in my fingers, the numbness hadn't bothered me"—when she asks her husband to caress it for the first time, she is shocked by how much she "hated the sensation—or rather, the lack of it—of being touched there" (120). "My new breast, on which so much time and money and hope had been expended, felt like dead meat" (120). When her husband touches her, Mayer is physically reminded that "this new appendage was breast-like only in appearance" (120). Her chest lost the basic bodily quality or sensibility that Merleau-Ponty has termed the "crisscrossing" of the toucher and the touched: "the interrelations of the inside and the outside, the subject and the object, one sense and another in a common flesh" (Grosz, *VB* 95). Mayer experiences the new breast as totally objectified, a bounded "appendage" bracketed and suspended from the normal corporeal experience of the intertwining of subject and object that, in Grosz's terms, "makes the subject open up to and be completed by the world" (96).

Her accumulating doubts about reconstructive surgery are further augmented when she encounters the sobering news about the potential risks of silicone gel implants. In 1991, a year and a half after her implantation process was completed, she decides to undergo another operation to exchange her implant with a safer model. This time, she is fully aware that she faces a number of surgery-related risks, from capsular contracture, scarring, and infection, to bleeding, skin necrosis, and displacement leakage or rupture of the implant itself. She also knows that "the implant would not last forever, that someday I would face another decision and another operation" (126). Although the reconstructed breast makes her clothes look better, she still finds herself wondering

if Audre Lorde wasn't right, and I long for what I imagine would be the clean, spare feeling of nothing but skin and muscle and ribs. My skin is numb beneath my arm and for a few inches on either side of my scar, across the entire front of the reconstructed breast. Although this would be the case without reconstruction, too, having the artificial breast there exaggerates this loss of sensation, stretching the area, and making it both more prominent, and more poignant, considering the location of this normally sensitive and erotic part. (123)

Indeed, not only does the artificial breast remain disintegrated from her "inner experience" (114), or body image, but it clearly enhances the sensation of bodily loss by physically making present—"stretching," "making . . . more prominent, and more poignant"—the absence of breasted experience. It is this persistent, lived experience of corporeally constituted lack, rather than an identification with a common political or theoretical struggle, that brings her, at the present tense of the narrative, to embrace Lorde's perception that "prostheses are often chosen, not from desire, but in default" (Lorde 65). Thus, she admits that "[w]ere it socially acceptable for a single-breasted woman not to wear a prosthesis in public, and were I able to do so without undue self-consciousness, there's no question in my mind that this is the choice that would feel more natural to me" (122).

Mayer's candid account of her lost sense of femininity as the decisive cause in her opting for breast reconstruction demonstrates the contiguous relationship between biological processes and cultural constructions. Her mastectomy, as she says "was only the last and final straw" (121) in the gradual accretion of related concerns, including infertility, hysterectomy, weight gain, aging, menopause—"each of which had some bearing on this basic issue of sexual body image" (120). Conversely, her experience of living with the reconstructed breast highlights the interconstitutive reciprocity between cultural constructions and personal embodied experience over time, which is clearly shown to have a formative role in establishing new awareness and knowledge. It is within such productive reciprocity, articulated in "the story of a particular affliction, as it has touched and altered a particular life" (Mayer 6), that a potential for transformative agency prevails. "Writing about my illness," Mayer says, "has provided for me a sort of armature upon which I can deposit, as a sculptor does bits of wet clay, the raw substance of memory and experience to form a new image, a new sense of who I am" (6). Apart from this salutary effect on her confidence and sense of self, her experiential account of mastectomy, chemically induced menopause, and breast reconstruction is important for feminist politics and embodiment theories not merely because it shows, once again, that women are culturally disciplined to identify their femininity with their breasts but also because it suggests that sexual self-image, what Mayer terms her "womanhood," has a lot more to do with biological and chemically induced processes and the way they click into the available normalizing cultural practices than many contemporary feminists are likely to accept.

Unlike Lorde, who refused to undergo chemotherapy and was spared the desexualizing effects of this treatment, Mayer had to struggle at once with her profoundly changed "sense of femaleness" and with the mystifying cultural constructions that led her to envision reconstructive surgery as "the single and magical cure" (121) for the loss of her sexual self. Consequently, while Lorde can celebrate the point where she resumed making love to herself after her mastectomy as the initial step toward her recovery (25), Mayer finds herself "living in a state of perpetual envy and longing—not for the ideal female form . . . but for my own lost self, as I used to be" (121). Despite their differing approaches to their postmastectomy bodies, however, both Lorde's and Mayer's accounts work to broaden the range of critical self-interrogation and self-reflection afforded to women with breast cancer. Their shared commitment to everyday experience—the conviction, in Lorde's words, that "first you hurt and then you cry" (41)—invokes an exploration of the practical and immediate demands of their embodied selves that considers the effects of institutional practices on personal experience and yet does not essentialize experience or make claims about the cultural constitution of *the* female experience or *the* female self.

What is at stake in these experiential accounts are the narrators' conscious responses to the situational, temporal, and interconstitutive personal and political effects of bodily practices within phallocentric society. Contemporary feminist criticism has yet to explore such concerns from a phenomenological perspective. The emphasis of feminist studies today on the subtle disciplinary modes that produce inescapably docile and usable bodies has replaced second-wave feminist inquiries into the pragmatics of women's experience and the emancipatory potential of their common embodied practices. Overly suspicious of any perspective that doesn't meticulously distinguish, first, between various *kinds* of women (Moi 8), feminist criticism neglects experiential accounts of women's specific subjection to normative definitions of how women's bodies should feel and look. The next section of this chapter will demonstrate that the fear of essentializing "women" or "women's experience" by pointing at shared embodied and discursive practices is unwarranted. In fact, the narratives of breast cancer I shall proceed to discuss indicate levels of sophistication and self-consciousness from which feminist embodiment theories can only gain.

UNACCOUNTABLE BODIES

In the last twenty years or so, adjuvant chemotherapy following mastectomy has become a common treatment for women with breast cancer. Regardless of the severity of their diagnoses and prognoses, women who write about their experience of breast cancer—evidently, in periods of remission—emphasize the onset of menopause as the result of chemotherapy as a taxing aspect of their life with the disease. "Breastlessness," says Christina Middlebrook, "is what the world seems to think that breast cancer is about" (178). Yet for her as well as for many other women, a far more difficult effect of treatment is to discover, as she says, that "my libido has gone south" (178). A professionally trained Jungian analyst, Middlebrook is forced by her experience of illness to retract her long-held convictions about the relationship between body and mind: "As a Jungian analyst, I did not have the capacity to believe that anything *physical* could tamper with, let alone *destroy* my sexuality" (182). In a chapter of her breast-cancer memoir called "The Secrets of Remission," she half-jokingly exclaims that she "would kill for estrogen" (171), fully aware that her situation is defined, rather, by the reversal of these terms: the very estrogen she craves "would kill [her]" (171). A similar recognition of the effects of treatment on her embodied self is voiced by Barbara Rosenblum in *Cancer in Two Voices*. Rosenblum describes her experience of menopause and

THE INVADING BODY

the absolute disappearance of all the physiological signs of sexual excitement following her fourth course of chemotherapy, remarking that this "physiological fact made me realize that the agreement and understanding I had with my body were no longer in effect" (157). Her ironic conclusion echoes Middlebrook's: "[F]or me," she says, "sex does not work in the head" (158).

Unlike Mayer and Lorde, whose narratives end optimistically with the remission of cancer, Middlebrook and Rosenblum tell the story of their struggle with advanced, metastatic—indeed terminal—breast cancer. Middlebrook writes a year after she completed a long process of treatment, including radical mastectomy, a failed course of enhanced chemotherapy supported by an experimental white-cell colonizer protocol and follow-on radiation, which was followed by yet more radiation and two more courses of chemotherapy, then blood pheresis to collect peripheral stem cells with a backup bone-marrow harvest leading to a successful bone-marrow transplant and the prospect of three years (or less) until the cancer will grow again (178). Rosenblum's book, which includes journal entries by her and her partner, Sandra Butler, traces a very similar protocol of treatment, except that she refused to undergo a bone-marrow transplant and had more courses of chemotherapy until it no longer worked. She died at home from complications of liver cancer at age forty-four. Rosenblum's and Middlebrook's stories are concerned with the experience of the sick body as a trigger and cause of a crisis of meaning that required them to radically revise their previously taken-for-granted agreements and understandings "with" and "of" their bodies. While their narratives, like Lorde's and Mayer's, discuss their altered bodies in terms of how they appear to others, their more urgent need is to demetaphorize both their illness and their bodies by exploring the various pragmatic and felt manifestations as well as the cognitive and emotional consequences of bodily collapse. Through writing about their experience of illness, they search for "a new language of the body," which, as Rosenblum acknowledges, is "the language of symptoms, not of sexuality" (159).

Since the 1960s feminist theory has concentrated on sexuality as a primary area of female embodiment that is culturally constituted and constrained but can also be subversive and even empowering.[16] The narratives of breast cancer this discussion explores occupy a space outside the variegated and ramified feminist discourse on the sexual body, which ranges from the dominant second-wave feminist distinction between sex and gender, to the continentally inspired celebration of *jouissance*, to the strictly constructionist view of the sexed body that paved the way for the more recent emphasis on the subversive/creative performance of gender identities promoted by queer theory. Terminal illness narratives do not consider the body in terms of pleasure and play, symbolic possibilities, or gendered "styles." They certainly do not view it as a wholly constructed locus of cultural signification, a position that, as Toril Moi has pointed out, places biological facts "under a kind of mental erasure" (42). Even when they raise issues related to body aesthetics, politics, and sexuality, they invariably ground them in the lived experience of idiosyncratic bodily limitations, losses, and pains. This does not mean that subjectivity in these texts is reduced to, or essentialized by, certain bodily features or biological facts. Rather, these narratives provide rich phenomenological resources for examining the complex relationship between subjectivity and embodied experience insofar as they textually enact Merleau-Ponty's concept of corporeality as embedded in subjectivity, or, as Grosz has defined it, "as the material condition of subjectivity" ("Bodies-Cities" 103).

Of paramount attention in each of these experiential accounts is the tense relationship between the lived body and the normative objectified body—that is, between the experienced, experiencing body and the seen, touched, medically treated, and culturally formed body. In normal situations, as Gail Weiss has argued, the body image, or corporeal schema, plays a significant role in mediating between lived and objectified bodies.[17] The body image, in fact, secures bodily stability by constructing, deconstructing, and reconstructing itself, from one moment to the next, in response to the continual changes in the body and in the situation (Weiss 17). This is not the case in terminal illness, where the situation of the drastically changing body overwhelms the body image's usual plasticity and ability to accommodate change. In terminal illness, as these texts show, the experienced boundaries of the body lose their normal correspondence to the topography of the internalized gestalts that form the body image. "I could not believe how rapidly my body shape was changing"

THE INVADING BODY

(162), Rosenblum writes. In her memoir, she desperately wishes to pin-point the experience of bodily disintegration and the devastating effects it has on her previous sense of the stability and predictability of her body.

> What is it like to live in a body that keeps on changing? It's frighten-ing, terrifying, and confusing. . . . It produces a slavish attention to the body. It creates an unnatural hypervigilance toward any and all sensa-tions that occur within the landscape of the body. One becomes a pris-oner to any perceptible change in the body, any cough, any difference in sensation. One loses one's sense of stability and predictability, as well as one's sense of control over the body. It forces you to give up the idea that you can will the body to behave in ways you would like. (163–64)

Rosenblum's journal validates theoretical insights about the role of body image in lived experience inaugurated by Merleau-Ponty and Paul Schilder and further pursued and refined by feminist scholars such as Grosz and Weiss. It also provides the unique perspective of an individual's conscious struggle to verbalize her experienced and experiencing body—paradoxically by underlining its resistance to interpretation and, indeed, to language. Although she uses a slightly different terminology than do Grosz and Weiss, Rosenblum's primary concern is to thematize the ways in which the experience of terminal illness and the effects of treatment undermine the body image's ability to maintain bodily stability and pre-dictability. The corollary of the loss of embodied coherence, she notes, is the disruption of the habitual, taken-for-granted skill of interpreting bodily sensations as messages.

When the sick body is insistently present, the individual forfeits her ability to interpret its signs. "Interpretations of bodily signals are premised on the uninterrupted stability and continuity of the body" (164), Rosen-blum says. However, with aggressive cancer, the body's boundaries and sensations change so fast that the body image, on which we rely for a "sense of where and how our body is spatially positioned as well as a tacit un-derstanding of what our corporeal possibilities are at any given point in time" (Weiss 17), is seriously affected. The body image's dynamic, recon-structive resources either lag behind, failing to accommodate the rapid physiological changes, or extend, as it were, in all directions to embrace the mass bombardment of sensations. In the latter case, the body image's very plasticity seems to belie its stability and, hence, its efficacy in constructing meaningful gestalts. "When you have cancer," Rosenblum says,

> you have a new body each day, a body that may or may not have a relationship to the body you had the day before. When you have cancer, you are bombarded by sensations from within that are not anchored in meaning. They float in a world without words, without meanings. You don't know from moment to moment whether to call a particular sensation a 'symptom' or a 'side effect' or a 'sign.' It produces extreme anxiety to be unable to distinguish those sensations that are caused by the disease and those that are caused by the treatment. Words and their referents are uncoupled, uncongealed, no longer connected. You live in a mental world where all the information you have is locked into the present moment. (166)

For Rosenblum, recovering embodied meaning depends on extricating her experience of illness from randomness and from the grasp of the present moment. Not only her body image but her very subjectivity seems threatened by the disappearance of recognizable embodied patterns that contribute to a sense of bodily continuity in time.

> Sensations come and go; they disappear for a while and they return; they change. They may add up to something, they may not. They may have meaning; they may not. I must wait until something else happens, until I have an accretion of evidence, until a pattern emerges, if I'm lucky enough to have a pattern. . . . And most of the time, I live in a world of random body events. I'm hostage to the capriciousness of my body, a body that sabotages my self of a continuous and taken-for-granted reality. (166)

It is by undertaking the task of learning "a new language, a new vocabulary . . . the deeper structure of [the body's] grammar" (165–66) that she attempts to circumvent the arbitrariness of body events and, thus, to restore temporal continuity and embodied meaning. "The patient's task," she says, "is to learn the new language, hoping that the body will remain stable enough" (166).

And yet, learning and sharing the new language of the body are not equivalent experiences. "The problem," as Rosenblum defines it, is that

> When I have sensations in my body, it's an unsharable experience; I become aware of the limitations of language in describing those sensations and thus relieving myself of their burden. I grow increasingly aware of the illusion of the intersubjective nature of the world. The world is shattered, language dissolves, and there is only body and its feeling. Even a private language, such as I have with Sandy [her lover], is a self-contradiction. There cannot be private language. Interactions slow down, collapse, lose their meaning and integrity. I observe myself trying to talk but am isolated in an imprisoned, solipsistic world, experiencing the terror, panic, and isolation because we believe in common language, common culture, common understanding. (129)

Rosenblum's experience of solipsism points to the contiguous relation between embodied patterns and linguistic constructions. Although not necessarily verbal themselves, the dynamic patterns that constitute the body image are shown, by negation, to enable accessibility to language and thereby also to interpersonal interaction. When experience is determined by "random body events," language, too, dissolves. Embodied alterity, the felt irreducibility of difference that does not lead to a coherent differing structure, drastically diminishes the usability and truth-value of institutional structures. The experiential gap between the sick person and the world, and its negative impact on interpersonal relations, can not be more clearly stated. However, precisely because it is stated in language, Rosenblum's solipsism is not complete, at least not insofar as her journal entries and reproduced letters to friends restore textual continuity and establish intersubjectivity through her audience's collaborative reading. At a later date, she explicitly acknowledges her commitment "to find words to apply to sensations I've never had before . . . to find meaning and stability despite a changing body" (167). Through the narrative of her experience of illness, and by consciously "experimenting with mood, voice, tone, and style" in order "to write things that moved the reader" (85), she has not only, however partially and transiently, overcome her crisis of meaning but also fulfilled her initial wish, on receiving the diagnosis of cancer, "to live self-consciously (and perhaps die self-consciously) in an exemplary manner" (13).

For terminally sick people, the loss of bodily coherence and stability diminishes communication through language and entails the loss of spatial forms of communication between bodies. Thus, the security that comes from a normally lived sense of analogy between our body image and the way our bodies are viewed by others is seriously reduced in sickness. Sick people can no longer relate to their bodies through identification and interaction with the projective healthy body. "I can't even remember what it is like to have a normal metabolism, normal energy, normal hair, and a normal body" (95), Rosenblum writes. When Christina Middlebrook asks her husband to take her photograph, which she intends as an obituary photograph that "will hang in the Jung Institute Library with the other deceased analysts" (161), it strikes her that she has no sense of how this portrait will look. "An obituary photograph is meant to show exactly who I was and what I looked like," she says. "But since cancer treatment, that image is a continually confusing one. I *do not know* what I look like" (161). The incident demonstrates cancer and cancer treatment's destruction of what Weiss termed "the intercorporeality of embodiment," explained by saying that "the experience of being embodied is never a private affair, but . . . always mediated by our continual interactions with other human and nonhuman bodies" (5).

For many cancer patients, encounters with other people with cancer in cancer groups, at hospital cancer centers, or on the street provide a necessary source of interactive projection and identification. Middlebrook recalls that once, when she was in treatment, and bald, she was driving with her husband through an intersection, and she "noticed that the driver approaching from the right had short, telling, chemo-curls. I snatched off my beef-eater hat and waved at her. When she saw me she tooted the horn, gave me thumbs up, grinned . . . I felt giddily victorious. I knew what my battle was, then. I knew what I looked like" (161–62). At the present tense of her narrative, however, her body image occupies a liminal, and limiting, intercorporeal zone. "Now," as she says, "my status is not so clear" (162). In remission, she "look[s] normal" to others, and, consequently, she feels "no longer entitled to reach out to strangers with bald heads" (162). But, then, "cursed with the knowledge of fate, of our vulnerability" (165), neither can she genuinely interact with the able-bodied.

Her suffocating sense of isolation—"I cannot breathe for the loneliness" (116)—is clearly a combination of failed embodied and verbal interaction with others. As she writes, this loneliness is intensified by the refusal of others, healthy people, to relate to the "knowledge of [her] foreseeable death" (99): "I never dreamed the difficulty people have finding a way to speak about cancer, serious illness, death. Sometimes others' need to minimize what has happened startles me" (133). The others' avoidance and denial of her situation underline not only the primacy of experience, expressed in the conviction that "[i]ntellectual understanding pales before experience" (194), but also shows the contiguity between embodied knowledge and a certain usage of language. Thus, "generations speak different languages. So do people with cancer. We use the same words but we must have different dictionaries. Things I say seem unintelligible to people who live outside the cancer realm. Certain of their phrases fall harshly on my ears . . . I guess that if you haven't been there, you just can't learn it. You can't get it from a book, or from interviews. You can only speak the language by living there" (122, 131).

"Then," she says, "miraculously, communications do occur. I speak. Someone understands" (131). These rare moments of understanding are what motivate her to pursue her attempt, in conversation and in writing, to communicate her "determination . . . to face what is coming, not to change it" (199). Fully aware that she "cannot overcome the unarguable fact that metastatic cancer is inevitably fatal" (199), she wants others to acknowledge and bear witness to her situation now, before she dies.

What I want is this. I want the well-entrenched American denial system to change. We are taught that when a person informs us "I am dying" or "I'm in deep shit here," we are to respond by saying, "Oh, no. No, you're not. You'll be fine."

I want a different response. I want interest and curiosity. I want the same concern I'd get if I said that I had been laid off from a job or had broken a leg. I want someone to say "God, how awful. How're you doing?" I want someone to ask, "What's it like?" (135)

Inextricable from the need for a witness, and a caring response, is the desire to impart the knowledge she has gained through her experience of cancer. Her illness narrative intends to answer the unspoken query "What's it like?"—for what she has learned through the experience of terminal illness is precisely that bodies are a source of knowledge. Her embodied experience has made her realize that the boundaries between the sick and the healthy are only temporary, provisional, and culture-bound. The task of facing death, the struggle to let go, awaits all of us. "For us cancer patients, that task just comes a little sooner. Some of us have skipped a generation or two. I, at fifty-three, speak comfortably about my body's decline with eighty-year-olds" (200).

Like Rosenblum and Wendell, Middlebrook insists that her knowledge of fate and vulnerability is not metaphorical but a lesson taught daily by the lived body. This kind of embodied knowledge is not equivalent to and cannot be learnt through conventional medical discourse. According to medical tests, she is in remission, yet her body's revolt against the lasting effects of treatment is a continual reminder that living with Stage IV cancer is all about endurance, never a cure. "Transplant pain is with me every day: bone pain, joint pain, foot pain, esophageal pain, headaches, ear-aches, jaw pain, edema pain, tooth pain, bruised shins, difficulty swallowing, difficulty eliminating, heart fibrillations, shortness of breath, fatigue, fatigue, fatigue" (165). The prospect of learning to live with bodily limitations and with the knowledge of imminent death is not helped by the medical system, which is oriented toward viewing the body as an object of knowledge rather than as a condition of subjectivity. "Medicine and high technology have not been adequate to the task of teaching me how to live, daily, with this disease. In no way has either helped me prepare for death" (192).

Conversely, the taboo that forbids speaking of death in polite society challenges the legitimacy and authority of her learned experience by confusing conventional speech about the body with knowledge embedded in the lived body:

Almost automatic words come out of our mouths to protect us from the reality of death when someone says she is dying.
"No you aren't," we protest.
"Don't talk that way!"
"Just think how lucky you are to _____." Fill in the blank [. . .]
Then there is, "You never know." I have struggled to find a response to "you never know." All I have come up with is "but, I do know," and that one makes me feel rude. (206)

The slippage between talking about the body and experiencing the complex life of the body, "much of which," as Wendell says, "we cannot interpret" (330), leaves the discourse about the sick body deceptively open to equally valid opinions and, subsequently, to the skeptic's condescending response to these opinions—"you never know." For Middlebrook, however, the skeptical and conventional responses of others merely reinstate the standoff between the sick and the healthy in terms of their respectively different usage of language—a difference, as her narrative affirms, that is contingent on concrete situations of differing embodied experience.

As with other taboos that confer magic power to words, the fearsome facts of degeneracy and dying are socially devalued through outright denial, conventional metaphors, or silence. Writers of illness narratives, therefore, negotiate between the aversion and nervousness their experiences evoke and their desire for a witnessing, compassionate audience. Middlebrook's strategy of negotiation is the unpacking of the mythical, false causality between voicing the inevitability of her early death and her embodied experience of dying. As she gently tells her avoidant sixteen-year-old daughter, "Talking about my dying . . . is not going to kill me. Not talking about it will not save my life" (31). Treya Killam Wilber similarly attempts to disengage her illness from the rigid, flattening hold of conventional metaphors by piling up the accumulating details of her

treatment: "tests and confusing results and conflicting opinion and difficult choices" (348). In a letter to her friends, she expresses her wish to ac-
tualize her experience of metastatic breast cancer, explaining, "I have included all these details . . . not because the numbers or the results or even
the choices I've made are important but because the details of the daili-
ness of living with this disease bring alive generalities like 'living with cancer is an emotional roller coaster,' . . . 'we can't plan ahead past next week,'
and 'this will go on and on until the end.'" (348). More explicitly, Musa
Mayer protests against the common, stereotypic tales of inspirational
heroism "in which the cancer patent [is] sustained by her faith in God and
her family's love" (73). These stereotyped stories, she says, "make us lose
touch with . . . the mundane, day-to-day feel of what it's like to encounter
the darker aspects of our human heritage—to live with disability, with
chronic illness, with despair and uncertainty, with the threat of impending loss of function and death" (74).[18]

While they fight conventional metaphors through the use of other
metaphors, supplanting stereotyped stories with other stories, all of these
writers are motivated by the certitude that, whatever the shortcomings of
their telling, the experiences they relate are real. "Real cancer is not a metaphor," says Middlebrook as she notices her own tendency to metaphorize
her experience through the language of war. "War is war. Cancer is cancer. Symbolic death is not death. The urge to soften them, to fend off their
reality, to metaphorize them, this urge overpowers our ability to speak the
truth" (203). Once more, it is important to realize that "truth" in these
narratives is never an abstract or absolute concept. Rather, it is the truth
of an irreducibly concrete, historically situated, experiencing and experienced subjectivity. Juliet Wittman writes in her breast-cancer journal that
you respond to the diagnosis of cancer "as the person you are—the product of a lifetime of action, thoughts and decisions, big and small" (56).[19]
Much like lived experience at large, the experience of a life-threatening
disease is an amalgam of lived conditions and choices, and, stark and ter-
rifying as the experience of cancer is, living with cancer does not essentialize the body, or entail only one way of conceptualizing the body or
writing about it. If anything, and in contrast to the monist, stereotyped

formulations of terminal illness in medical case studies and in the media, illness narratives strive to textually enact the irreducibility of the experience of illness. "Simplification," says Rosenblum, "maybe that's what this process is called. It feels more like coming into one's fullest and truest self and simply acknowledging what is. . . . Although Heidegger is not my favorite philosopher, there are now lessons to be learned from him. A dog dogs. The world worlds. Barbara Barbaras" (127–28).

The phenomenological perspective of illness narratives considers writing about the body as a commitment to the situated nature of embodied subjectivity, "the process of committing what I experience and what I learn and the way I am challenged to paper" (Wilber 348). While feminist constructivist theories are inclined to break down the body into an "objective" and a "subjective" component, which roughly correspond to the categories of "sex" and "gender" (Moi 73), writers of illness narratives are engaged in investigating the dynamic interaction between their changed bodies and their sense of self. Because they attend to the situated particularities of the experiencing body, they respond to the question of "what is it like" in ways that render irrelevant the gulf between epistemological concepts of objectivity and subjectivity. Even when they are trained academics, fluent in feminist and deconstructive discourses, these writers rely on their immediate, everyday experience of illness to check, reconstruct, or confirm their subjectivity.

Thus, Eve Kosofsky Sedgwick accentuates the felt discrepancy between her lived experience of breast cancer and "the formal and folk ideologies around breast cancer" that construct the disease as "the secret whose sharing defines women as such" (262). In her essay "White Glasses" she acknowledges that "[in] the day-to-day experience so far of living with and fighting breast cancer . . . I feel inconceivably far from finding myself at the center of the mysteries of essential femaleness" (263). Like Mayer, who relies on her experience of illness when she criticizes the stereotyped stories of breast cancer, and Middlebrook, who warns against the use of symbolic language that evades the reality of living with cancer, Sedgwick uses her experience of illness and cancer treatment as a way of grounding her skepticism in respect to the purportedly essential traits of embodied identity and their determinist correspondence to social categories such as gender, race, and age.

She comments, thus, on "the dizzying array of gender challenges and experiments [that] comes with the initiations of surgery, of chemotherapy, of hormone therapy":

> Indeed, every aspect of a self comes up for grabs under the pressure of modern medicine . . . That pretty, speckled, robin's-egg blue pill with the slightly sinister name "Cytoxan"—it was developed during World War II as a chemical warfare agent; when, as per doctor's instructions, I drop four of this "agent" into my bloodstream every morning, the *mildest* way to describe what is happening is via the postmodernist cliché that I am "putting in question the concept of agency"! I have never felt less stability in my gender, age, and racial identities, nor, anxious and full of the shreds of dread, shame, and mourning as this process is, have I ever felt more of a mind to explore and exploit every possibility. (263–64)

The postmodernist and deconstructive convictions Sedgwick voices about the self are in full accord with her embodied experience. In fact, it is her experience of cancer treatment that particularizes and enforces for her the sense of the inherent instability of the self, advanced by postmodernist theories and values. That she uses her everyday, lived experience of breast cancer in order to dismantle the cultural aphorisms that construct breast cancer as "the secret whose sharing defines women as such" exemplifies the way corporeal and discursive knowledge intersect in the situated perspective of the embodied subject. Like other experiential accounts of illness, Sedgwick's account serves to identify the experience of living with illness as an extreme test-case situation that highlights such normally concealed, interrelated dialectic conditions of lived experience as biological processes, body image, and institutional historical and cultural constructions.

In insisting on the idiosyncrasies of their particular embodied experience in specific situations, writers of breast-cancer narratives may significantly contribute to feminist theories of embodiment. On one hand,

THE INVADING BODY

breast-cancer narratives extricate the body from the allure of abstract conceptions of pure, unreachable ("objective") materiality, but on the other hand, they also resist the grip of the reified and reductive equivalence of the body with sexuality and sexual differences—constructed or otherwise. As my discussion of mastectomy and breast reconstruction has shown, even the central question of sexual body image is contingent on concrete situations of embodied experience of alterity in illness. These concrete situations, in turn, generate specific political demands for social change that should directly affect embodied identity. As Lorde has said in an earlier quoted passage, the fact of being "[s]urrounded by other women day by day, all of whom appear to have two breasts," makes it very difficult "to remember that I AM NOT ALONE" (61). For Lorde, as well as for the other writers whose texts I have discussed, embodied alterity is a key experience in the concrete reality of living with breast cancer, both for the sick individuals and for "certain other people" who suppress the existence of, say, one-breasted women because in this way "they do not have to deal with [the sick] nor themselves in terms of mortality nor in terms of difference" (Lorde 64). However, unless we wish to argue that one-breasted women form a whole new gender or, indeed, sex, breast-cancer journals clearly reveal that embodied alterity can hardly be grasped primarily in terms of sexual differences.

The phenomenological perspective of experiential accounts of terminal illness makes abundantly clear that attending to the dying body or to the body in pain compels an engagement in the complex interrelation among specific conditions of embodiment that may include but are never restricted to sexual differences and sexual oppression. Such an engagement may prove methodologically productive for the study of "normal" processes of embodiment, since, while it discloses the cultural base of inferiorized group identity, it avoids "the culturalist traps of the disappearing body" (Marshall 65)[20] that occur when the experienced and experiencing body is conceived of as a mere reflector of social practices and discursive processes. The crises of meaning breast cancer and other illness narratives detail often point to the sick body as a catalyst for attaining a revised outlook or learning to affirm a new sense of self. This does not mean that the body is rendered as an "objective" or a "natural" arena or ground in which an existential crisis occurs or on which a new subjectivity is superimposed.[21] Attending to the experience of illness in these texts identifies, rather, the interconstitutive relations between bodies and subjectivity and the particular embodied consequences these relations bear for individuals in specific social and historical contexts.

3

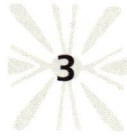

CONFESSING AIDS

IN *THIS WILD DARKNESS: THE STORY OF MY DEATH* (1996), HAROLD Brodkey examines his decision to disclose his experience of having AIDS as a form of truth telling or confession, which he upholds against the social expectation that it is generally better to lie about such things.

The overwhelming powerful thrust of bourgeois life is to lie, is to hide things. A house, an office, is a stage set. I think that much of what is hidden is chosen arbitrarily, family by family, person by person. Having secrets and confessing them is what *deep* attachments are about. Telling the truth is never wholly recommended, however. And now this. You might live longer with AIDS than you're supposed to, medically speaking, by not telling anyone you have it. . . . With AIDS, one is told, assuming the stress of public excoriation on top of the stress of the disease itself—which is, if you will, a state of precariousness beyond belief—is probably unwise. . . . If you lie and deny that you are ill, the lying helps you live—helps you keep fighting. . . .

I'd rather be open about AIDS and scoff at public humiliation than feel the real humiliation of lying. I'd rather try to make this a death as much like any other as I can. (114–15)

This passage conveys the complexity of the decision to discuss one's experience of terminal illness, which, in the case of AIDS, is horrendously magnified by the multiple and often contradictory discourses that influence the construction and significance of AIDS and shape our response to the people who have it.[1] Telling the truth about having AIDS is only apparently parallel, as Brodkey acknowledges, to disclosing any other secret in bourgeois society. Unlike the common secrets of families and individuals, which Brodkey believes to be "chosen," however "arbitrarily," "person by person," the secret (rather than the fact) of having AIDS is culturally multilayered. It is a secret that imposes a collective as well as an individual identity and whose telling, moreover, may adversely affect one's physical well-being in a fundamental way.[2] Thus, if in normal middle-class life, "[h]aving secrets and confessing them" is perceived by Brodkey as a mode of behavior that enhances interpersonal intimacy—it is "what *deep* attachments are about"—the confession of having AIDS carries a much more complex relational value. With AIDS, the possibility of normalizing the experience of terminal illness, of "mak[ing] this a death as much like any other as I can" by deepening interpersonal attachments, inevitably engages the sick person in an attempt at self-explanation and self-justification that must address the overwhelmingly negative cultural constructions of the disease. To "tell the truth" in this context and "scoff at public humiliation" is no mere rhetorical gesture but a risky commitment that testifies to the interactive relations between bodies and cultural representations.

Brodkey's strangely overlooked autobiography stands at the center of this inquiry.[3] His posthumously published book is composed of diary entries in essay form that convey his response to his HIV-positive condition and his awareness of his imminent death, covering the period from his first hospitalization, in spring 1993, until late fall 1995, two months before he died. The fact that the essays were originally serialized in the *New Yorker* during the years of Brodkey's illness invests them with a sense of poignancy and urgency, which is complemented by his precise, rhythmic prose. The result is an extraordinary document that combines the immediacy of testimonial truth with the self-reflexive, diamond-hard lyricism of a modernist poet. As in many other illness autobiographies, the authorial stance here seeks to construct a coherent story out of severe bodily ailment. This is achieved in part through the conventional master plot of illness narratives, which extends chronologically, from the narrator's detection of minor symptoms of the disease, through tests, diagnosis, hospitalization, medical treatment, and partial recovery.[4] More pertinently, though, Brodkey uses the convention of writing about the experience of illness as an existential turning point around which he constructs an interpretation of his life before he became ill and presents a rich mode of living with terminal illness in the narrative present, as "[m]y life has changed into this death, irreversibly" (17).

Significantly, this last act of self-writing is distinguished from the autobiographical fiction of his past. Unlike his career-long—and, some would say, obsessive—endeavor to employ autobiographical materials as the building blocks for his fiction, Brodkey's illness autobiography demands to be read as personal testimony.[5] The motto preceding the book's title reads: "I don't see the point of privacy. Or rather, I don't see the point of leaving testimony in the hands or mouths of others." In defining, thus, *The Story of My Death* (the book's subtitle) as personal testimony that disregards the conventions of privacy in polite society, Brodkey has aligned himself, deliberately or not, with other contemporary writers of terminal illness narratives, whose personal accounts attempt to convey their own truth about the embodied experience of dying.[6] Granted, his last work employs a narrative style and narrative strategies that recall his autobiographical stories and novels. Like his much-praised collections of short stories, *First Love and Other Sorrows* (1957), *Women and Angels* (1985), and *Stories in an Almost Classical Mode* (1988), and the two long-awaited and less-well-received novels, *The Runaway Soul* (1991) and *Profane Friendship* (1994), his illness autobiography includes personal memories of adolescence and maturity. It, too, engages the themes of childhood, growth, sexual experimentation, and parenthood. Furthermore, it employs the unique narrative style that Brodkey has used since the 1980s and that has, in singular fashion, played with complex syntactical structures and sudden shifts in place, point of view, and time.[7] However, while in the autobiographical fiction, the thematic concerns and narrative strategies served Brodkey's purpose of representing the subtle and elusive procedures of memory, in his illness autobiography, he is directly focused on the experience of illness in the narrative present. Both the familiar themes and the narrative style are recruited to confess, justify, and explain not only the truth about the experience of bodily collapse but also the emotional hurdles of cultural stigmatization.

Cultural stigmatization and its correlative feelings of shame, victimization, and abjection, and the humiliation that accompanies the exposure of terminal illness, is by no means restricted to people infected with HIV. In a society where health is upheld, paradoxically, both as a normative, regulating category and as an ideal state of personal utopia, the decision to disclose a seriously debilitating illness is itself transgressive, verging on admittance to a state of sin.[8] Both bodily manifestations and talk of physical deterioration are an unforgivable affront to polite Western society. Indeed, we aspire to hide even biological signs of aging that only remotely imply senescence and the progression toward death, whereas medical research itself, as Bateson and Martin note, "has traditionally dodged the question of the evolutionary significance of senescence, and has looked for a cure as though immortality were an option" (34). How, then, are we to reconcile such an overwhelming reluctance to admit the experience of physical decline with the commitment to be open about one's disease expressed by many personal narratives of terminal illness? How, in other words, may writers such as Harold Brodkey overcome the audience's profound resistance to the "old story," as one reviewer of an illness narrative has put it, of "one more trip among inhuman and/or saintly doctors and nurses, one more chronicle of personal failure, personal triumph"?[9]

My purpose in this chapter is to show the centrality of the confessional mode to Harold Brodkey's autobiography of terminal illness. Brodkey's text will serve to demonstrate how narratives of terminal illness may adopt the textual practices of the confession as a way of negotiating the cluster of negative associations and feelings that surround and govern our culture's response to the experience of terminal illness and, by way of metonymy, towards the terminally ill. It is important to realize that Brodkey uses the confessional mode ambivalently, both in earnest and as a literary ploy. Thus, in spite of his desire to "be open about AIDS" (115) as the hallmark of normality, his equation of AIDS with a fatal secret and the

THE INVADING BODY

analogy he draws between truth telling and confession transform his experience of terminal illness into the language of sin. As we shall later see, his autobiography is strewn with evidence of his internalized abjection—his sense of being contaminated and "thoroughly repellent" with sickness (97). And yet, his employment of the confessional mode can be seen, alternatively, as a way of resolving the tension between his desire to normalize the experience of dying and his awareness that dying from AIDS is always already constrained by the particularly oppressive cultural metaphors of AIDS. By manipulating the power relations that structure the confession, Brodkey subverts the authority of the public constructions of AIDS shared by his own audience. On the one hand, he conforms to the traditional structure in which the person confessing reveals his or her transgressions to an authorized audience, the confessor, hoping to achieve purgation or reconciliation through the audience's understanding and forgiveness. On the other hand, he consciously exploits the highly charged contents of his confession as a means of undermining his audience's resistance to conventional illness stories. In this way, I contend, he is ultimately able to express his personal, embodied truth of terminal illness, which, as we shall see, stands outside the restricting public discourses on AIDS.

In analyzing Brodkey's confessional narrative, I concur with Paul Ricoeur's view that the power relations inherent in the confessional mode are neither stable nor static. In *The Symbolism of Evil* Ricoeur remarks that the confession capitalizes on the audience's need to understand at the same time that it "excites attention by its very character as scandal" (8). This ambivalent rhetorical manipulation of audience has inspired Dennis A. Foster to identify the confessing sinner as "both penitent and tempter" (17). People who write about their terminal illness are indeed scandalously free to transgress social codes of polite behavior, for instance, in concentrating on the details of physical disintegration that accompany their illness. The confessional mode enables writers of illness narratives to thematize their sick bodies—albeit at the cost of casting their audience in the role of confessors. Thus, in tempting their readers with the allure of power that comes with the authority to judge the confession, say, as a test of character, writers of illness narratives can extend their appeal beyond the particular, "natural" audience of other people at risk.

This view of the confession as an ambivalent rhetorical mode differs from the currently dominant approach to confessional texts in cultural and autobiographical studies. In the last twenty years or so, it has become a critical commonplace to treat confessional narratives as inevitably caught up in a network of power relations that create (constitute) the confessional subject and shape (regulate) his or her confessional truth. This strong constructionist approach derives from Michel Foucault's theory of confession in the first volume of *The History of Sexuality: An Introduction,* even though Foucault himself, in volume three of *The History of Sexuality,* which he wrote as he became ill much later in his life, added nuances to this radical position. In *An Introduction,* Foucault repeatedly emphasized that although to confess is to engage in a reciprocal practice in the sense that both the confessing subject and the confessor participate in the production of confession, the very form of confession is so "thoroughly imbued with relations of power" that it renders the speaker's truth a mere "shimmering mirage" (60, 59). Rather than express individual truth, the confession both requires and shapes truth according to internalized, self-regulating conventions that define, for confessor and speaker alike, "what is most difficult to tell" (59). The person confessing, that is, has been stripped by Foucault and his followers of his or her traditional agency—of the privilege of speaking freely and independently—while the confessional truth has been likewise exposed as a product of socially hegemonic discourses. In every confession, as in any autobiographical text, what we find instead of personal truth is a mirror image or a reproduction of social authority.[10]

Foucault's view of the self, or rather the subject, as constituted through power relations in the confessional act has had an enormous influence on autobiographical studies. In spite of disclaimers—Susan Bordo qualified Foucault's theory of power and knowledge as a description of social relations rather than a recipe for reading texts (*Essays* 295)—since the 1980s, critics of the autobiographical mode have continually drawn on Foucault's theory of confession as a way of redefining the connections between text and context, poetics and politics. Thus, an important critic, Leigh Gilmore, postulates that autobiographical truth in general "has less to do with [a] text's presumed accuracy about what really happened than with its apprehended fit into culturally prevalent discourses of truth and identity" (*Autobiographics* ix).[11] Foucault's enabling contribution to our understanding of the emerging subgenre of illness autobiographies examines the historical and social processes by which the religious notions of error or sin, excess or transgression, were translated into medical categories of the normal and the pathological. Undoubtedly, after Foucault, we have become more alert to the ways in which cultural institutions and discourses, in this case religious and medical discourses, control and regulate social practices, such as confessions of sins and personal accounts of illness.

And yet, by focusing exclusively on one moment in the development of Foucault's rich thought, the strong constructionists among literary and cultural critics canceled out the possibility of the subject's intentionality and, with it, also the related concepts of individual agency and resistance.[12] The implications of this view for the reading of illness narratives cannot be overstated since it effects the denial of the sick person's agency in speaking of his or her experience of illness. According to this view, what makes confessional illness narratives so compelling is that the authority of confession as a culturally dominant discourse of truth telling converges both with the social authority of the medical establishment and its "scientific" formulations of diagnosis and prognosis; and with the traditional authority of religious rite, especially of deathbed confessions, including the judicial legacy and symbolic weight attributed to one's last words. Still, a major concern in this chapter is my apprehension that strong constructivism, which attends primarily to the political dimension of cultural discourses of this kind, seriously impoverishes our understanding of illness narratives and the experience of coming to terms with illness.

Countering the discourse-based view of confession as "a rhetorical process of assimilation of the transgressive into the normative" (Bernstein 32), I am interested in the sick individual's attempt to negotiate between the ways illness is felt and the cultural narratives constraining it. Accordingly, I ask whether we can treat writers of illness narratives as authoritative agents in spite of the cultural discourses that frame the truth of their accounts. The following reading of Brodkey's illness autobiography, therefore, will first describe the means by which the confessional mode not only frames his account of illness but also colludes in and reinforces our culture's particular metaphoric constructions of AIDS. This part of the analysis will show that the confessional authority of the public discourses on illness exposes the agency of the sick person's account as a delusion. However, in the second part of the discussion, I will emphasize the ways in which the confessional structure paradoxically also gives the writer license to recall the sick body in terms of embodied experience instead of as a textual construction, a metaphor. My argument will be that the strong constructionist view of the confession fails to account for the writer's sense and expression of embodied experience, and thus, it becomes morally complicit in our culture's marginalization and silencing of the terminally ill.

Readers familiar with Brodkey's autobiography realize, of course, that the revelation that he has AIDS is not the only confession in his text. The narrative is organized around two major confessional plots: that of Brodkey's discovering the disease and his ensuing struggle with it, told in the narrative present, and that of having been sexually abused at the ages of twelve and thirteen by his stepfather. These two seemingly unrelated confessions are in fact causally connected by Brodkey, so that the extended period of incestuous abuse and the conditions that effected and terminated it are presented as an explanation of—indeed as a catalyst for—his contracting HIV much later in life. Significantly, the autobiographical details that accompany the confession of sexual abuse are not there as an end in themselves but serve to validate the interchangeable causality between illness and sexual transgression. This is not a reconstruction of "a life story" in terms of what it can now be seen to have been (as can arguably be said of the autobiographical stories collected in Brodkey's *Stories in an Almost Classical Mode*) but a thematic packing of the zones of illness, crime, guilt, and punishment from which the narrator extracts explanatory insights that help him understand the experience of illness in the narrative present tense.

Illness frames the confession of sexual abuse, serving the double function of motivation and excuse. Not only were Brodkey's adoptive parents seriously ill at the time of the abuse, but their illness vindicated, for the young Brodkey, both the assaults themselves and his parents' enthusiastic celebration of the abuse as a passionate "love story" (58). "[T]he major drama of my adolescence," says Brodkey,

> was that my adoptive father, Joe Brodkey, who was ill with heart trouble (a handsome invalid, as one would write in pornography) assailed me every day for two years, sexually—twice a day, every morning and every evening, when I was twelve and thirteen. He had nothing else to do, really. He was ill. . . .
>
> I confessed nothing. I complained to no one. My mother, herself ill with cancer and drugged, warned me oracularly, "If I were you, I'd learn to keep my mouth shut." I don't mean to be insulting to her memory, but she was excited, even inspired by the situation, which—it took no great brains to see—helped keep both her and Dad alive: it interested them, this *love* thing (58, 59).

Illness, therefore, in the text's logic, is responsible for the abuse as well as for Brodkey's silent acquiescence, which he understands as having helped keep his ill parents alive. Conversely, when Brodkey as narrator finally confronts his stepfather and puts an end to the assaults, his resistance marks his apparent transformation from victim/healer to abuser/patricide, for he becomes convinced that in resisting his father, he has virtually murdered him.

> Then, I killed Joe Brodkey. But I didn't know—scientifically—it would kill him to talk to him with intelligence and finality. I stood up and leaned against the bureau and he lay on my bed, and I said he could not touch me any more at all, not even a handshake, unless he *behaved*. Murder is always an experiment in reality by the poor, proud mind. Rhetorically and emotionally it was enough to condemn him. (141)

Following this avowal of guilt, the causal connection Brodkey proceeds to draw between the circumstances of the abuse and his present condition with AIDS is quite straightforward. As an adult, laden with the awareness of having been a traumatized child and with the overwhelming burden of patricide, he "experimented with homosexuality to break my pride, to open myself to the story [with Joe Brodkey]" (61). Then, "[a]t the end of the period in which I pursued the 'truth' of these matters, I met a young schoolteacher named Charles Yordy," (141) whose biography (he was also an adopted son) resembled Brodkey's. Significantly, what attracted him to Yordy and triggered their relationship was a felt analogy between his lover's relation to his sick stepfather and his own "story with Joe Brodkey" (142): "Charlie had been adopted, and he was nursing his dying father. . . . It isn't that I saw myself in him. No. But for the first time I glimpsed bits, portions of my story with Joe Brodkey in another person's life" (142). Years later, Yordy dies of AIDS, and, as Brodkey dryly suggests, "I think he was the one who gave it to me" (143).

The chain of events that Brodkey constructs, then, builds causal and temporal connection among analogous narrative sequences containing illness, homosexual relations, and death, each causally patterned itself. Sexual abuse, propelled forth by his parents' illness, is directly related by Brodkey to his adult experimentation with homosexuality, which is seen retrospectively as an attempt to explore, reconstruct, and comprehend the "story" with Joe Brodkey. More particularly, of course, this exploration of sexuality led to the relationship with Charles Yordy that has effected his dying from AIDS. From this perspective, too, his present terminal condition is experienced as retribution for his guilty refusal to continue fulfilling his father's sexual needs "even though he [was] dying": "He [Joe Brodkey] accursed me. Now I will die disfigured and in pain" (60, 61).

However, the persistent element that pervades these events, and that psychologically and politically redefines the relation Brodkey constructs between the two major confessional plots in the text, is yet to be discussed. The underlying cause for his illness, according to Brodkey, is indeed moral but also innate: it has to do with his being "cursed with irresistibility," an inherent, morbid sexual attractiveness he claims to have had since he can remember himself as a baby, and that has since governed his life and "partly determined my death" (56, 55). As Diana E. H. Russell observes, the notion of being "cursed with irresistibility"—the belief that one has innate powers of seduction—is common among sexually abused children, especially among children abused by a close family member. It

THE INVADING BODY

is instilled in the abused child as the result of a projection of the abuser's sexual feelings on the child, and of the child's subsequent internalization of the abuser's accusation that the child is, in fact, the seducer.[13] From this psychoanalytical perspective, the transformation, noted earlier, from Brodkey's sense of himself as a traumatized child to owning that he had murdered his father—from confessing crimes committed against him by others to a confession of his own criminal act—is misleadingly incomplete, since it leaves out his confession of guilt for his father's sexual assaults, namely, "my long history of boring irresistibility" (59).

In retrospect, this history means that "[f]rom infancy, my life has always been, always, always, on the verge of my being eaten alive: *I could just eat you up.* In my childhood, people talked a great deal about me and quarreled over me—and threatened force. And there was violence, some of it directed at me" (54). Being "cursed with irresistibility" means that "I cannot find in memory a day in my life without some erotic drama or other" (56, 57–58). It also means that, even after "the drama, the persecution" of incest has ended, "such assaults, such oddities, comic and manic, or melancholy or dangerous, occurred everywhere, as if by contagion— with the football guys, with old friends, with the mothers of friends, with strangers. I was even half-abducted once, forced into a car, but I fought and talked my way out of it" (59–60). In other words, Brodkey's feelings of victimization and guilt significantly precede his resisting, and thereby "killing," his father. Rather, they stem from his sense of his own omnipresent, deviant irresistibility defined as an inherently transgressive identity trait that attracts and compels sexual violence. Evidently, while such recognition of his own culpability partly absolves his step-parents of their collusion in the abuse, it works to intensify Brodkey's own guilt for condemning his father. Irresistible, and thus morally implicated at the core, he can hardly blame others for the sexual transgressions committed against him, and he therefore "deserves" to feel guilty for condemning his father and, by the same token, to be accursed with AIDS.

This sense of intrinsic depraved irresistibility—the same irresistibility that granted him "undeserved welcome" in the insiders' social circles of New York "off and on for the last forty years"—mobilizes the constellation of negative structures of illness, sexuality, guilt, and death that frame the confession of sexual abuse and explain the infection with HIV in terms of cause and effect (57). Ironically, even as he tries to break the causal connection between sexual identity and illness by probing beyond his babyhood—into his biological mother's life and death—the alternative explanation he offers for his contracting AIDS reiterates and confirms his innate sense of sin. In this alternative, cyclic account he sees himself as "being part of an endless family story of woe and horror," in which his "being accursed" with AIDS is a repetition of his real mother's illness and death from "a curse laid on her by her father, a wonder-working rabbi" (95, 94). Just as his mother was accursed with terminal illness for betraying her orthodox father, Brodkey feels accursed for his betrayal of her, for rejecting her on her deathbed and for "clinging instead" to his healthy stepmother:

> When I was barely two, she died painfully, over a period of months, either of peritonitis from a bungled abortion or from cancer, depending on who related the story. Then Doris, my father's cousin, and Joe came for me and, later on, adopted me. I was told that Doris took me once to the hospital to see my mother, who smelled of infection and medicines and that I refused her embrace, clinging instead to the perfumed Doris; the rescued child was apparently without memory of the dying mother. (Perhaps that was the real crime, and not my obduracy with Joe.) (94–95)

Significantly, the "real crime" of refusing his mother's embrace is not remembered but instilled in him through diverse "family accounts" (94). Even the nature of his mother's illness remains ambiguous, its superimposition of cancer and illicit sexuality evoked through the gap between the two versions of her illness story. Just as the cause for his mother's illness "depend[ed] on who related the story," so Brodkey's own sense of a cyclic repetition of guilt, his "mood of being accursed, of being part of an endless family story of woe and horror" (95), is revealed as a product of his adoptive family's mythology, which is itself constructed out of halfrumors and mystical insinuations. Perhaps, as Paul de Man claimed of Rousseau's *Confessions*, there is no guilt prior to its mechanical produc-

THE INVADING BODY

tion by language (299). Yet, the shifting causes of guilt in Brodkey's illness narrative—from his condemnation of his stepfather, to his acknowledgment of his own innate moral blemish, to his doomed participation in his family's endless "story of woe and horror"—persistently point outward, to familial and cultural narratives that define fatal illness, in Susan Sontag's words, "as a test of moral character" (41).

Poststructuralist criticism such as Foucault's allows us to question Brodkey's confessions of guilt as well as the self that confesses its guilt, and to attribute both the guilt and the urge to confess it to discursive mechanisms that precede the individual and are nonetheless internalized as one's most cherished and private notions. Such mechanisms include our culture's deeply entrenched homophobia, which results in varying degrees of overt and covert internalized homophobia among both bisexuals and homosexuals.[14] From the perspective of the homophobic mainstream culture, AIDS is a gay disease, one that, as G. Thomas Couser notes in *Recovering Bodies*, "reduces the individual to his sexual identity and condemns him to an early death from a harrowing illness" (87). Indeed, most people's response after learning that a person has AIDS is "to determine the degree of responsibility (or culpability) of the person affected" (Couser, *Recovering Bodies* 86). "Myths of identity," adds Thomas Yingling, "*have framed* the interpretation of AIDS, and it remains a disease that attaches—rightly or wrongly—to identities: gay, IV-drug user, African, hemophiliac, infant, transfusion patient (the 'guilty' and 'innocent' 'victims' are labeled through some category of identity that promises—falsely—to explain their contraction of the disease)" (303). Our culture's obsession with "the moral cause" of HIV infection and with the "proven" guilt of gay and sexually promiscuous victims, who are seen as criminals deserving punishment, has caused AIDS patients to internalize the idea that they themselves bear the responsibility for having contracted the disease—a belief incorporated, literally, from the same cultural mechanisms that police homoerotic desire. Already regulated by the discourse of marginality, gays who have AIDS are prone to internalize the very mainstream, dominant interpretation that isolates and stigmatizes them as the Other.

Thus, although at one point in the narrative Brodkey asserts the commonplace medical knowledge that "AIDS is not phallocentric, not homocentric, not picky in the least about its carrion" (43), the confessional structure that dominates his autobiography consistently conflates his contraction of AIDS with his own previous—if not innate—sense of transgression and guilt, for which his illness is seen as punishment. Furthermore, feelings of shame and abjection dominate his telling of the experience of having AIDS: "No one can explain what it means to be marked out"; "I must admit I felt truly accursed"; "being ill is like the experience of public nakedness in dreams"; "[t]he aura of punishment is simply present" (48, 94, 124, 44).

In a way that reinforces the interconstitutive cultural constructs of sexual identity and terminal illness, the text juxtaposes another set of culturally prescribed values that center round Brodkey's relationship with Ellen Schwamm, his wife. From the perspective of a Foucauldian critique, Ellen represents an assembly of normative, healthy, "decent" bourgeois practices. Literally and figuratively, she acts as Brodkey's rescuer—first, from his homosexual past, and, second, from the self-hatred and humiliation of dying from AIDS. Brodkey sees Ellen, whom he introduces in the text as "my human credential," as the obvious antithesis to his depravity: "People think she is good-looking and trustworthy and sensible, whatever they think of me" (8). Their elopement and more than fifteen years of marriage embody a clean break with the past: for Brodkey, meeting Ellen marked the end of his promiscuous homosexual experimentation, whereas Ellen "left her husband for me. She walked out on everything. No one backed her but her children" (14). Both of them had to live through years of "public attacks that were a bit on the vicious side" (14). Ellen, especially, "was pretty generally pounded after she ran off with me"—"she had met everyone who had been in my life in the years before her, literary and ordinary and homosexual. None of them accepted her. Not one" (61).

As has been noted with regard to the instrumental function of autobiographical details in the confession of sexual abuse, the relationship with Ellen, too, is not presented as an end in itself, but serves to highlight her crucial role in Brodkey's AIDS confession. Self-assertive and disciplined in the face of public attacks, Ellen becomes a full-fledged partner in Brodkey's confrontation with "the humiliation of dying—humiliation in regard to the world" (91). Her vigilant and "omnipresent" competence at comforting—which is "the governing element of any household she runs, any love affair she is in"—earns her a share in the experience of illness to the extent that even Brodkey's doctor relaxes his professional notions to include her in "what was best for me; he saw it more and more in terms of us, of Ellen and me . . . he began to tell her what I should do medically, and I could close my eyes and rest while he did it" (15, 85). At once his nurse, lover, "omnipotent angel," and "omnipotent mother," Ellen epitomizes, through her conduct during the course of his illness, such values as generosity, sensitivity, competence, and "as-if superhuman" feminine unselfishness, which are implicitly contrasted with the behavior characteristic of the exploitative relationships that informed Brodkey's life before their marriage (120, 116). Her "as-if inexhaustible tenderness . . . far stronger and more unflagging in effect than any courtship intensity that had ever been directed at me," is identified with healthy and life-giving resources that mitigate Brodkey's overwhelming sense of being "accursed and diluted," "filthy with AIDS," "mostly pain and odors, halting speech and a sick man's glances" (96, 118, 97).

The confession of how it feels to be sick with AIDS thus branches according to the traditionally Catholic dual meaning of confession: the confession of transgressions and the confession of faith. On the one hand, Brodkey confesses his feelings of utter helplessness, desolation, and shame at being "marked out" by AIDS (48). On the other hand, he confesses (praises, celebrates) the tenderness and innocence of his rejuvenated relationship with his wife, who vows to him that his illness is "one of the happiest times of my life" (98). Back at their apartment after his two-month hospitalization for *Pneumocystis carinii* pneumonia,[15] Brodkey testifies of his wife's devout nursing in terms of idyllic courtship: "my arrogant deathliness and her burning gentleness were dancing together in a New York light in our apartment. This was like childhood, a form of playing house" (96). In a reversal of traditional gender roles, Ellen is the savior-prince who "decide[s] to wake [him]" (97) with a life-giving kiss:

A kiss—how strange her lips felt, and the quality of life in them . . . the heat of her skin, the heat of her eyes so close to me, everything in her was alive still and full of the silent speeches that life makes . . .

I accepted her and her affection as truth, as being as much truth along those lines as I was likely to want. This meant that by the second week I was home we both realized that, in this limited world of mutual watchfulness and of unselfishness-for-a-while, this period was for us, in awful parody, honeymoonlike, and that this was acceptable to both of us, grief or death at the end or not. (97–98)

Confessing, that is, celebrating, Ellen's love as sufficient truth, a truth that is as real in its "silent speeches" as the "savagery and silence" of sickness, becomes a source of strength and self-confidence: "I came alive again, for a little while. Well, why not? . . . You still pass as human among humans" (98).

We have seen that the text's two major confessional plots identify the condition of terminal illness as a curse or punishment for a dynamic constellation of primarily sexual transgressions. By contrast, the confession of faith in the marriage upholds the healing, indeed humanizing, power of such normative constructions as heterosexual love and wifely devotion. The narrative thus conforms to what Steven Dansky has termed, following Foucault, the binary system of licit and illicit created by the medicalization of sexuality as the locus of pathology (38). Brodkey's free and nonjudgmental talk of his past homoerotic experiences blurs the boundaries between licit and illicit desire only superficially. The direct links the narrative constructs between illness, sexual abuse, and homosexual orientation, and between homosexual experimentation and dying from AIDS, embed homosexuality in a scandalous confessional sequence in which homosexual practice originates in exploitation and leads to terminal illness and imminent death. Moreover, Brodkey's sense of an inherent personal blemish, his "cursed irresistibility," intensifies the connection between his sexual identity and a persistent element of moral depravity that mobilizes the negative constructions of illness, sexuality, and death noted previously. In the confession of how it feels to be a person with AIDS, these negative constructions continue to operate, culminating in a sense of "final castration" that identifies the disease with self-erasure and ultimate punishment (6). In contrast, the celebration of his marriage to Ellen introduces a countersystem of normative discourses on sexuality and illness that works to restabilize the privileged status of heterosexuality as healthy and life giving, a humanizing force. Hence, homosexuality is further foiled and objectified as something less than human, interchangeable with identity erasure and a deadly pathology.

It might be said, then, that this reading of Brodkey's confession as the productive effect of regulatory power in the Foucauldian sense cancels out the confessing subject's authority and agency in controlling his illness story. Consciously or unconsciously, he is compelled to reiterate the culturally dominant constructions of discursive legitimacy. And yet, this reading overlooks Brodkey's painful awareness of the formative discourses that frame every discussion of AIDS. More pertinently, it excludes his attempt to negotiate between such awareness and the novel, devastatingly physical sensation of bodily disintegration and violent loss of his familiar, healthy self. It is important to recognize, however, that the lived experience of illness is messy, rarely adhering exclusively to unified models of illness, of either cultural or biomedical construction. The incongruity between how illness is experienced and how it is formulated disrupts the constitution of the confessing subject as fated to repeat and reflect the power relations inherent in the confessional mode. Brodkey's mode of resisting the culturally dominant constructions of AIDS will be discussed shortly in terms of intersubjectivity. For now, I would like to examine the implications of his very different struggle with the medical formulation of his illness, that is, his conscious attempt to express the embodied experience of illness as standing outside the "objective" medical knowledge of AIDS as disease.

Brodkey's representative of the medical establishment is Barry, his doctor, who not only urges him to define his condition according to the medical model but also insists on the clear-cut link between the medical construction and the meaning of AIDS:

Barry insisted that I be clear in my mind what having AIDS means . . . What I think he wanted me to know is that AIDS is the terminus in a thus far fatal viral infestation, which was identified in 1981–82 and arbitrarily, perhaps not finally usefully, defined to conform to surface symptomology. Roughly, this means that when you have AIDS, you're hospital material. The terminology is distinctive: you will die of "complications from AIDS." Babes and old geezers are special prey to the stubborn murderer *Pneumocystis*. Whoever you are, your biological identity now occupies a thin cage with prowling, opportunistic diseases. (43, italicized in the original)

Notwithstanding today's much more optimistic biomedical construction of HIV infection, the point here is that Brodkey's reiteration of the medical formulation of AIDS as "the terminus in a thus far fatal virus infestation," and his depiction of the "biological identity" of people with AIDS as in "a thin cage with prowling, opportunistic diseases," evoke and converge with the sense of doom and abjection raised by the cultural metaphors of AIDS. Brodkey clearly recognizes the connection his doctor wants him to make between the medical model of AIDS and his own "biological identity," but in making the connection he also invests it with significance drawn from the cultural constructions of illness.

This seemingly unavoidable blend of cultural and medical meaning-making is circumvented, however, by Brodkey's suggestion of another mode of tending to his embodied experience of illness. Thus, says Brodkey, "I am inside an experience that the doctor cannot share from the inside, yet the reports he gives me and the actions he takes at a given moment are the only real source of news I have about myself" (43). The quotation manifests Brodkey's awareness of the constructive, indeed materializing effects of medical authority and intervention. Nonetheless, while the material reality of the experience of illness is formulated by medical reports and actions, it also remains outside medical discourse, forming, in Judith Butler's words, "an ontological thereness that exceeds or counters the boundaries of [here, medical] discourse" (8). In other words, Brodkey's awareness both of his dependence on medical authority for the sake of making sense of what he experiences, and of the loss of the sense of an autonomous self that such dependence entails, does not annul the presence of the body that is experienced as alien to medical hegemony as well as to the lost healthy self.[16]

The sick body demands an articulation that exceeds the boundaries of cultural, medical, and existential constructions and is induced, as Drew

THE INVADING BODY

Leder has claimed, by the body's "own episodic temporality of rally and relapse, which makes it stand out from the amorphous time of health" (81). What is excluded from the paradigm of regulatory discourse is the embodied knowledge of being so sick that "[e]verything [is] suffocation and the sentence of death," with "all sense of presence, all sense of poetry and style, all sense of idea . . . gone" (Brodkey 11). The experience of physical disintegration defies discursivity, even though, once it is formulated in discourse, it is inevitably reconstructed in a way that constitutes material reality as "an *effect*" of discursive procedure (Butler 30). Retroactively, the experience of critical illness is posited by Brodkey as a condition in which "nothing was a phrase or seed of speech, nothing carried illumination in it, nothing spoke of meaning, of anything beyond breath" (11). This is an experience of cognitive void and temporal-spatial contraction along the lines of Elaine Scarry's formulation of extreme pain as self-, world-, and language-destroying. "As the content of one's world disintegrates," says Scarry, "so the content of one's language disintegrates; as the self disintegrates, so that which would express and project the self is robbed of its source and its subject. World, self and voice are lost" (35). Once more, writing about one's illness evidently reconstructs and integrates the experience of illness into available discursive frames, and is, thus, in a crucial sense not only formative but also antithetical to that experience. Yet, in a paraphrase of Butler's proposition of the formative power of discourse, to claim that verbal communication is formative is not to claim that it "originates, causes, or exhaustively composes that which it concedes" (10). Rather, the experience of unmediated pain continues to haunt the narrative's discursive boundaries of memory and loss as their "constitutive 'outside'" (8). In attempting to negotiate between embodied, cultural, and medical knowledge, Brodkey's narrative thus constitutes the experience of terminal illness in terms of the duality Butler has referred to as "that which can only be thought—when it can—in relation to . . . discourse, at and as its most tenuous borders" (38).

The construction of individual agency in terms of embodied experience defined as "a constitutive 'outside'" evades and, thus, disrupts the constricting paradigm of regulation and assimilation differently imposed by the cultural structure of confession and by the medical model of AIDS.

Moreover, besides this negative conception of agency, the text asserts the possibility of recalling the sick body positively, in terms of intersubjective experience. Intersubjectivity is achieved once the crisis of dying compels Brodkey, momentarily, to reify and relinquish his belief in the self as the hero and author of one's life story. "The trouble with death-at-your-doorstep," he says, "is that it is happening to you."

> Also, that you are no longer the hero of your own story, no longer even the narrator. Barry [his doctor] was the hero of my story and Ellen the narrator. The tale was of my death amid others' lives—like a rock in a garden . . . My private code, the actions of my past, what I had done, what had been done to me, all that was a physical and finite pattern now . . . I was a remnant of life, homeless psychically. (68)

In this state of "all present tense," of a psychic "stillness" that "represents a sifting out of identity and its stories, a breaking off or removal of the self," the notion of self-blame and the sequence of moral responsibility for his illness are also abandoned (40, 24). Physical collapse banishes previously held concepts about one's identity, "private code," and self-reliance, but at the same time it enables him to recognize that he lives, literally and emotionally, through interdependence on others. Thus, "my not caring if I lived or died hurt Ellen. And I was grateful that I could indulge my cowardice toward death in terms of living for her" (12). Living "for her" is soon replaced by living through her, either literally ("if Ellen was there" . . . "[t]he medicine came on time, the IV was properly adjusted") or psychologically: "I lived through Ellen's will from time to time during those days. I had her agility and subtlety vicariously. I had that merciful depth of her female self at my disposal. It was like that as long as she was awake, anyway, and as long as her strength held out" (45, 33).

Brodkey's stereotyped characterization of Ellen's "merciful depth of . . . female self," though obviously oblivious of fifty years of feminist criticism, should not be confused with the substantial, and to my mind sincere, depiction of the bond between them. Read in the "all present tense" context of dying, Ellen's sensitive care—itself dependent on her embodied ability to be strong and "awake"—exceeds its previously discussed signification as a representation of the privileged discourse of heterosexuality. The pragmatic appropriation of her health and "will" by Brodkey is not caused or exhausted by viewing it as a product or projection of cultural discourses. Cultural constructionism of this kind altogether overlooks what Terence Turner has defined as "the plural aspect of the body as a relation (both physiological and social) among bodies, rather than the singular and individual aspect of the body as the subject of sensations of erotic pleasure or pain" (44). That Brodkey needs Ellen and Barry in order to survive, that he sees them as the narrator and hero of his story, would be received as a mark of psychic homelessness only as long as he—and the readers—continue to equate the body wholly with its private, individualistic aspect. Once it is reified as "a physical and finite pattern," this private aspect of his illness story is no longer serviceable in reconstituting himself as a subject in process (68).

Intersubjective experience, by contrast, allows him to construct new cognitive paths that refamiliarize him with his past:

Take the matter of thought, of trying to think: I used [Ellen's] will, her sense of coherence if I wanted to comprehend anything. And—literally—I hadn't the strength to finish a thought without her help; it took two of us to carry a thought. She guessed at my purpose and knew my old thoughts about the nature of the world and my style, and she patched things together for me. And, as she began to tire in the circumstances of hospital treatment and the ailment, I became more sharply crippled. (71)

The embodied aspect of such interdependence is highlighted here through the direct relation between Ellen's lapse of energy and Brodkey's sense of becoming "more sharply crippled." Yet the converse contingency also occurs. To reread a previously cited passage, when he learns to accept Ellen and her affection "as truth, as being as much truth along those lines as I was likely to want," he can pursue his life in the following period of relative recovery in light of the gains of intersubjective experience: "There are things that have to be done, family things, literary stuff, things having to do with AIDS. I do them with [Ellen's] marks of interest and amusement on my face" (97, 98).

What such a rereading demonstrates is the reductive force of viewing confession only as a set of inherent power relations asserted as an all-embracing maxim. By focusing on confession exclusively as a discourse of power, strong constructionism mistakenly presumes that the political regulation of the sick body is the only tenable discourse on the body, one that focuses on the body as a conceptual object of discourse and thereby rejects any attempt to recall the body in terms of material action and intersubjective experience (Turner 44). Granted, Brodkey's text provides abundant evidence of the cultural and political production of the sick person's identity as a confessional subject. Yet a critical consensus that reads the confession as a priori antagonistic to the possibility of the subject's authority and agency would inevitably conclude by affirming the same self-evident truth from which it had started. In the case of illness narratives, this reading ends paradoxically by collaborating with the stigmatizing social mechanisms of control that dehumanize and marginalize the ill as voiceless Others. By treating the confession of humiliating bodily illness as the product of hegemonic, disembodied cultural discourses, cultural constructionism in fact denies the truth-value of the sick person's embodied experience and knowledge. In addition, strong constructionism is unlikely to accommodate the possibility that a sick person who is a professional writer, like Brodkey, may intentionally employ the confessional mode as a subversive rhetorical practice aiming to undermine his audience's resistance to terminal illness stories. The one-sidedness of confessional authority not only discredits the confessing subject's self-awareness but occludes any attempt at subversion or manipulation of a culture's policing or management of personal experience.

Viewing the confession as a dynamic rhetorical and collaborative act, however, allows us to account for a gradient of awareness and adherence to consensual thought that implicates the confessional subject as well as his or her audience. From this perspective, the confession is shaped by the image of the specific audience/confessor the person confessing has in mind—in this sense conceding the authority of regulating discourses asserted by cultural constructivism—but also, crucially, by particular audiences of readers who are themselves embedded within social and conceptual frames. The construction of a coherent confessional sequence that connects Brodkey's sexual identity with AIDS would, accordingly, depend both on the concept of confessor the narrative projects and on the concrete reader/confessor who may or may not commit herself to accepting, and thereby constituting, the unifying causality of such a confessional sequence. Furthermore, viewed in terms of a collaborative performance, the confession of terminal illness permits the reader to situate herself not only epistemologically but also emotionally and ethically. She can go beyond asking whether the confession describes or constructs personal truth, whether "there are facts outside of discourse or discourse creates facts and truths" (Phelan 15). Instead, a reading may center on empathetically tracing the textual slippage between cultural narratives and embodied knowledge, highlighting the complex relationships between bodies and discursive representations, but crediting, too, the sick person's attempt to negotiate and express the discrepancies and interaction between the physiological and social aspects of terminal illness.

An ethical response to confessions of terminal illness aspires to suspend and counter the reader's inclination to distance him- or herself from another person's confession of pain and humiliating symptoms either by reducing the confession to a mere story about the sick body or by treating it as the product or textual projection of cultural narratives about the ill. It may instead encourage an understanding of the ways in which one's response colludes in and reinforces the unifying, abstract coherence of such cultural narratives at the exclusion and sometimes erasure of the primarily concrete circumstances and embodied experience of the person confessing.

A striking passage near the end of Brodkey's autobiography—an extended analogy for his apprehension of imminent death—may prove instructive in signaling to the audience how they might try to approach his confessional text:

> At one time I was interested in bird-watching, and I noticed that
> when I saw a bird for the first time I couldn't really see it, because I had

no formal arrangement, no sense of pattern, for it. I couldn't remember it clearly, either. But once I identified the bird, the drawings in bird books and my own sense of order arranged the image and made it clearer to me, and I never forgot it. From then on I could see the bird in two ways—as the fresh, unpatterned vision and the patterned one. Well, seeing death nearby is very like the first way of seeing. (109)

Brodkey's bird metaphor acknowledges the interaction between culturally constructed patterns and our "sense of order" that mutually "arrange" and constitute what we know. Yet it also raises the possibility of a "fresh, unpatterned vision," which Brodkey claims to hold onto alongside the culturally constituted perception. While the problematic of looking "through" the identifying, determining cultural patterns is not resolved by Brodkey's formulation of the "unpatterned," his "first way of seeing" may nonetheless posit an implicit injunction for a modest, self-conscious mode of reading his, as well as others', confessions of illness. The freshly seen bird and the analogous "death nearby" both subsume and surpass prevailing cultural constructs. They are paradoxically both seen and incapable of being seen without help from the formal arrangement of received conventions. Similarly, as we try to approach illness narratives from an ethical viewpoint, we may want to remind ourselves of the importance of not erasing the validity of the narrated experience of illness, even though, like "the first way of seeing," the persistent reality of the writer's embodied knowledge continues to elude both our innate need for clarity and the integrative cultural patterns we recruit as a way of representing and conceptualizing it.

4

FLESH-TINTED FRAMES

IN THE PAST TWENTY-FIVE YEARS OR SO, THE COMPLEMENTARY
beliefs that photography offers a mythic, neutral window on the world
and that photographs can serve as transcripts of reality have been called
into question.[1] Against the common-sense understanding of the actual
and factual dimensions of photography—its ability to cut into visual reality by recording a certain moment in time—stands the prevalent critical
awareness of the photograph's constructed composition, which significantly undercuts photography's claims to objectivity or even verisimilitude. Professional photographers have always known that the photographic image is thoroughly constructed and permeated by language or
other cultural grammars. Since the late 1970s cultural critics have drawn
attention to the photograph's denotative elements, those aspects of the
photographic image that relate analogously to the reality "out there," as
mere effects of photographic treatment (the codified patterns of framing,
lighting, blurring, perspective), the selective organization of subject matter, and the mechanical apparatus of the camera itself.[2]

Constructionist criticism of this kind, however, fails to account for autobiographical illness photographs' concrete investment in specific temporal sequences beyond their formal frames. I argue that the testimonial
force of these photographs is better explained by attending to the dynamic processes of photographic production and reception, which shift

the evidential force of photography from the subject of the image to the viewer's sense of time. Exploring this shift is especially productive in examining the unique power of illness photographs to evoke both our understanding of their coded messages and our incongruent notion that the suffering they convey is real—not only in the sense that "this is how it was" but also in grasping that the time elapsed since a given photograph was taken matters crucially to the people in the photograph. Our knowledge that people with terminal illnesses are physically, and often visually, wasting away compels the viewer to reconstruct and project the images in illness photographs onto both the future and the past. Furthermore, the shock of recognition that usually attends our awareness that the author of an illness narrative we have read is dead seems even fiercer in the case of photographed self-portraits. Autobiographical illness photographs, then, are interesting not simply for their visual thematization of the sick body but because they test the current critical consensus about the medium of photography as wholly manipulated by arbitrary visual signs. They question the logic of the common critical claim that because the reality effect of photographs is inevitably constructed by signs, those signs must have no indexical connection to the reality toward which they point.[3]

This chapter and the chapter that follows propose to identify autobiographical illness photographs as an emerging subgenre of self-documentation whose indexical relationship with the reality of illness has the power to question the dominant critical assumption that there is a clear-cut separation of photographic representation (what we see in the picture) from prephotographic reality (what was there when the picture was taken). Like the illness autobiographies, yet in a different modality, autobiographical illness photographs foreground the concrete, sentient body as caught up and positioned among the cultural constructs and representational practices of terminal illness. The illness photographs that I examine vacillate between the boundaries of construction and contiguity in ways that parallel the vacillation of illness narratives between narrative construction and narrative contiguity with somatic experience. On the one hand, they consciously endeavor to produce staged, dramatized, images of illness, but on the other hand, they contain indexical references to the experiential reality of the sick subjects that they portray.

THE INVADING BODY

The following discussions of autobiographical works by Jo Spence and, later, in chapter 5, of those by Hannah Wilke, will analyze the inter-constitutive, dynamic processes of photographic production, reception, resistance, and exclusion as fundamental means by which these photographs either accentuate or attempt to disguise the tension between the indexically contingent and the previsualized and planned. In focusing on the tension between the staged and the real, I do not claim, however, that the relation between construction and contiguity in these photographs is necessarily symmetrical. On analysis, the constructed elements become far more distinct or extractable than the indexical marks of disease— partly because the photographers I discuss acknowledge their work as art, and partly since one of the persistent qualities of the photographic literal message is that it actively resists translation into language. These two chapters will place emphasis, therefore, on the paramount role of the audience in both establishing and resisting the photographs' truth-value. This is not a naive or superstitious return to the idea of photography as either mimetic or magical but an attempt to account for the paradoxical constellation of construction and contiguity that is the hallmark of even the most consciously postmodern of illness photographs. The photographs, thus, make even clearer what we have already seen in illness narratives: the mutual constitution of the reality of illness by discursive constructions and somatic experience.

Both Spence's and Wilke's illness photographs have attracted recent critical attention, particularly for their psychoanalytically invested treatment of dying. Thus, Jo Anna Isaak praises the artists' "last laughs" and "joyful utilization of the real" (49, 67), arguing for their similar performance of primary narcissism. By contrast, my own focus is on the range of interaction the photographs enable between artistic construction and contiguity with lived experience. In accord with my emphasis on close analysis of particular examples of self-documentation of illness rather than on applying a body of theory to case descriptions, I defer the theoretical angle of my reading to the second half of the following chapter. My method is twofold: first, I wish to analyze the experiential reality that the photographs represent, which includes political, social, and personal meanings; and second, I intend to show that these photographs' indexicality, their relation to the experiential reality they seek to convey, emerges at the levels of their production and reception. Disregarding the popular notion that most photography is the result of quickly taken snapshots, Spence and Wilke view the process of producing photographs as a complex, temporal, and interactive realm. Thus, in the process of making the photograph, the artists employ self-documentation not as an end in itself but as a reference point for conceiving other images of illness. In the process of reception, alternately, the audience's concrete response to the exhibited work compels, at the same time, both further revision and the creation of new images. Thus, it is not enough to explore the artists' treatment of illness or the finished "work" when seeking to detect the means by which illness photographs disclose as well as construct personal experiences of illness. The complex intersections of the performing subject, the viewers, and the invasive circumstances of illness must also be considered.

Jo Spence's prolific and variegated work on cancer is particularly useful to my project and will occupy a major part in the discussion. From being first diagnosed with breast cancer in 1982, through her second struggle with the leukemia from which she died in 1992, Spence engaged in an exploration of the relationship between issues of self-representation and self-construction and the cultural and political practices that effect the representation of illness. Moreover, the development of her photographic and written documentation of her experience of illness depends directly on the processes of production and reception that I am interested in. Spence's prolific and eclectic work defies easy classification, yet it may be retrospectively identified as an ongoing skeptical play with the conventional boundaries between the inside and the outside, the private and the public, and the personal and the political, themes that are more closely investigated after her breast cancer was discovered in 1982. Her diversified career as writer, teacher, political activist, and, of course, photographer is chronicled in her posthumous collection of essays, interviews, and photographs, *Cultural Sniping*.[4] For the purposes of this chapter it will suffice to roughly divide the trajectory of her career into two directions: her early ideological and political (Marxist-feminist) work in the 1970s; and the work on identity, subjectivity, and mental and physical health that be-

THE INVADING BODY

came her focus in the 1980s. The major shift between the 1970s and 1980s is a movement from a critique of "external" reality and its class, gender, and race inequalities carried out from the position of an independent observer to a representation of the artist's own position as a resisting subject who is nonetheless constituted, and to a large extent contained, by cultural institutions and practices. The second period, extending from the exhibition Beyond the Family Album (opened in London's Hayward Gallery in 1979) through her experiments with phototherapy and phototheater in the second half of the 1980s, stands at the center of the present inquiry. In terms of methodology, Spence intensified her use of techniques of previsualization and photomontage as a way of questioning the tradition of photographic realism, to which she added an exploration of personal materials—photographs, memories, her own and others' bodies—that she constructed as sites of individual and cultural interception.

Much of her new interest in this period in challenging the culturally constructed boundaries between the public and the private followed her health crisis in 1982. But this was not just a temporal coincidence. Her illness motivated an ultimate break from the critical-educational Marxist work in which she had been engaged for a decade. As indicated by The Cancer Project photographs,[5] the break was not an abrupt decision but stemmed from a gradual recognition of the inadequacy of the old methodology and theory, a recognition that depended on the personal experience of illness. Spence has testified that she initially meant to pursue her previous socialist-feminist agenda. When her breast cancer was diagnosed, she furiously resolved "to document the procedure of being 'processed' through the hands of the medical profession" (CS 130).[6] Her experience in the hospital as a powerless patient thus triggered an attempt at documentation that built on her earlier ideological work on the representation of working-class women and racial minorities.[7] As she later recalled, in taking "the three hundred or so pictures"—"thirteen rolls of film"—in the hospital, she acted out her sense of rebellion against her feelings of being out of control "coupled with a powerful anger" (CS 130–31).

The photographs she took then of the ward rounds of the consultant (figure 1, The Consultant's Ward Round) depict the hospital as a workplace, consciously emphasizing it as a social structure that dictates cer-

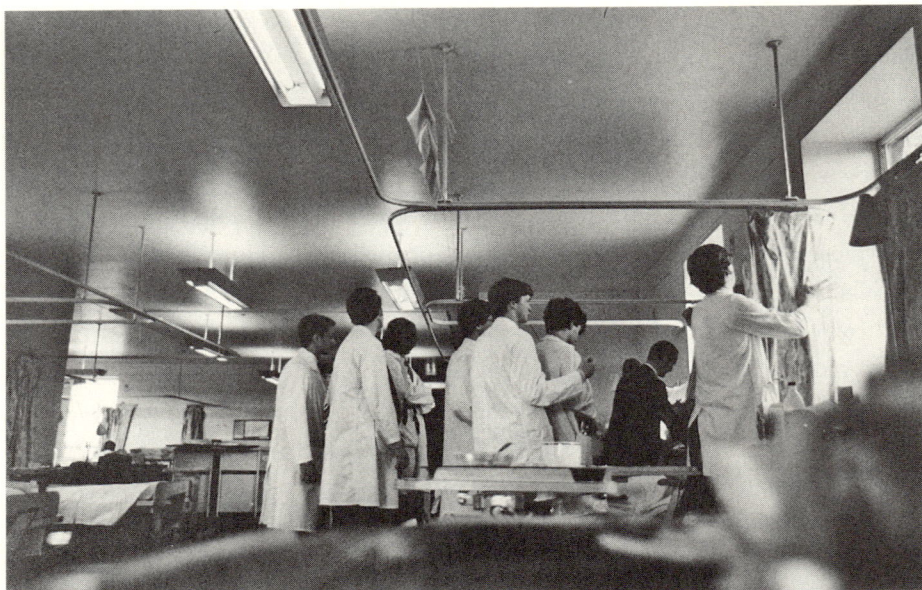

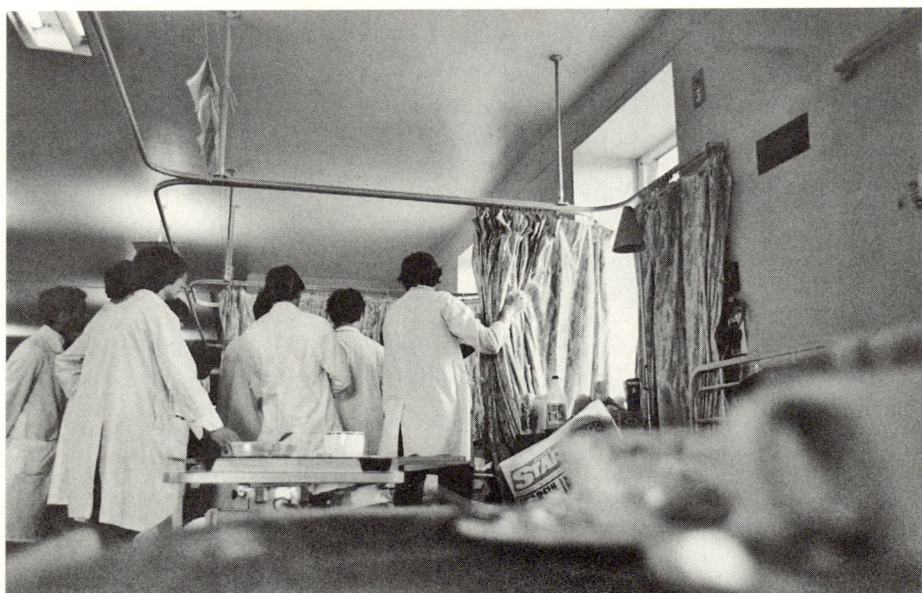

Figure 1. Jo Spence, *The Consultant's Ward Round.* 1982. From The Cancer Project, Nottingham. "He enters the ward dressed in an expensive suit and is surrounded by a flock of white-coated students. When he gets to my bedside I immediately stop taking photographs." (Courtesy of the Jo Spence Memorial Archive)

tain power relations between different classes, races, and genders. The workplace setting is suggested by the low angle of the camera, which magnifies the bright neon lights and the iron curtain railings hung from an overbearing ceiling. The hierarchical relation between the consultant and his attending students (all male) is marked by the difference in their clothing. However, the patients (all female) themselves are invisible or appear only from a distance; their presence is only metonymically traced by objects: beds, empty dishes on a night table, a protruding tabloid (a telling signifier of class). If there is a relationship between doctors and patients here, it is constructed through evident oppositions: the doctors are pictured as acting subjects while the patients are designated by still objects; the doctors are visually present, embodied, while the patients are altogether absent; the doctors are all middle-class men while their breast-cancer patients are (implicitly working-class) women. This set of oppositions clearly frustrates an idealized conception of a hospital ward as a humane place that is oriented toward the care and healing of the sick. The emphasis on patients' objectification and anonymity goes with the grain of theories of socialist realism, such as those of Georg Lukács, Bertolt Brecht, and Roman Jakobson, which analyze economic relations in capitalist society and their effect in obliterating people's individuality.[8] Accordingly, although in figure 1a a student is busy drawing the curtains around the bed of the patient who is about to be examined, figure 1b sequentially implies that, since the patient has been visually erased anyway, this act is more protective of the consultant's privacy than that of the invisible patient.

As a photographer, Spence's own position here follows her early educational practice of the subversive detection, exposure, and denouncement of social institutions in the tradition of documentary photography. Yet the critical distance and political empowerment that are usually associated with such a practice are here undermined and rendered transient and inconsequential by the reality of her own illness. What is missing from the above reading of the photographs is an indication of Spence's position not as a social activist but as a suffering patient. Indeed, the fact that she took the photographs from her own hospital bed turns the low angle of the camera into a contingency rather than the seemingly informed choice that helped to construct the suggested analogy between a hospital ward and a workplace. Years later, in 1990, Spence reconstructed the experience of taking these photographs in the hospital in words that highlight her emotional and political vulnerability at the time.

> Later, when I looked more carefully at the three hundred or so pictures I made, I saw images of the consultant's ward rounds on the morning I was to hear my diagnosis, followed by a picture (taken by my setting the self-timer and putting my camera on top of my locker) of my naked breast marked up for amputation. I then remembered that the entire consultation had taken less than five minutes. For me, this series represented moments of terror and a complete loss of dignity and power, followed by repressed rage at the ways in which I was silenced—professionally 'managed' from asking questions about my fate. (*CS* 131)[9]

The terror, the humiliation—the intensely personal experience of loss of power and dignity—are clearly absent from the previous reading of these photographs as a social critique. (The self-portrait with the marked-up breast is a singular exception that will be discussed separately.) For all the possibly productive effects of exposing doctor-patient relations in terms of power and powerlessness, visibility and invisibility, and subject-object dichotomies, the rigid ideological framework postulated by this critique excludes Spence both as subject and as author of her physical and emotional experience of illness. Even the rage she acknowledges to have felt has been repressed and rationalized. The caption retrospectively added to the photographs conveys Spence's sense of the shortcomings of this mode of "realistic" documentation. It reads: "The consultant's ward round. He enters the ward dressed in an expensive suit and is surrounded by a flock of white-coated students. When he gets to my bedside I immediately stop taking photographs" (*CS* 107).[10]

The caption calls into question Spence's photographic control of the situation. Its obvious understatement—"I immediately stop taking photographs"—resists the reality effect of the ward photographs by proposing what they fail to represent: Spence's coercion into silence by the superior power of the medical establishment. Five years later, in a keynote paper delivered at the first National Conference of Photography, she referred to the production of these photographs as a personal, and professional, turning point. Documenting the hospital setting, she said then, had prevented her from showing "how I was situated within that as a powerless patient, how I knew so little about my body that I had internalized my subjugation to the medical profession, or how the medical profession came to have the power of life and death which is rarely questioned" (CS 106–7).[11] Realistic documentation, although it helped her to assume momentary control, proved inadequate in sustaining her need to be seen as a human subject. It failed, too, as a methodology that might have helped her come to terms with her experience of illness by asking questions instead of reiterating the already known. "When I came out of the hospital," she has said,

> I needed to do research and to turn to theory to understand the essence of the political power of the medical profession. I then needed to seek for other ways of representing that reality which, eventually, involved the staging of personal tableaux for the camera. In this way I was able to produce photographs which helped me to ask questions, rather than to appear to give answers. (CS 107)

Yet before research and theory paved the way to staging herself as "a symbol, a metaphor for the many others in the same position" (Dennett, *The Cancer Project*, n.pag.), the self-portrait she made in the hospital of her marked-up breast already points in the new direction she was about to take. This is the photograph she mentioned in the passage quoted earlier (CS 131), and which she later titled *Marked Up for Amputation* (from The Cancer Project, figure 2). It was taken a moment after a doctor walked up to her on the hospital ward and marked her breast with a cross saying "this is the one that is coming off" (Evans 242). Spence faces the camera half-naked—and because she had to lay the camera on top of her locker, at chest level, her marked breast dominates the image by its sheer size and commanding whiteness. It is as big as her head, but credible, real. The viewer's eyes revert to Spence's exposed body parts, the whiteness of which is amplified by the dark red of the bed curtain and the darker blue and green of her dressing gown. The eye travels upwards from the white breast to the white neck and head and down again to the white hands. With one hand she lightly holds her dressing gown to cover the unmarked breast, the other hand clutches and resolutely pulls the gown to expose the other breast. Her resolution is reflected also by the tensed chin and strained corners of her mouth. However, the contrastive position of the hands—one relaxed, the other in a fist—reveals the difficulty of the exposure.

The image appears at first to have visually reversed the power relations implicit in the "consultant round" photographs. Here, the camera is introduced into the patient's zone, within the protectively drawn bed curtains. It displays her not only as visible and embodied but as an agent able to determine and control her own level of exposure. Nonetheless, although the doctors are absent, they have neither been erased nor dethroned of their position of supreme power. Their metonymic mark—the cross on Spence's breast—is clearly more than a sign; it is even more than a speech act. Rather, it should be defined as a body act, a physical branding that indexically, and at once, initiates, points at, and entails amputation. This is very different from the metonymic relations between the invisible patients and pieces of ward furniture implicit in the consultant-round photographs. There, metonymy was construed as a forensic device, representing the different social status of doctors and patients in the photographs' present tense (within their given frame). By contrast, the mark on Spence's breast is indexically tied with events that exceed the photograph's frame: it retrieves the past, the act of branding by an invisible hand, and, inevitably, compels the viewer's realization of the crucial future consequences of this body act. Ominously, the power relations between doctors and patients have been reinstated even more forcefully than before, since the asymmetry here is rephrased not in formal terms of visual presence and absence but in terms of imminent pain and the already determined bodily deformation. The collapsed categories of time that construct the photograph's meaning render the doctors as acutely present as the marked-up patient. However, the testimonial power and agency implied in the act of self-representation suggest an oppositional force that is congruent with Spence's explicit desire to use the camera "as a third eye, almost as a separate part of me . . . ever watchful: analytical

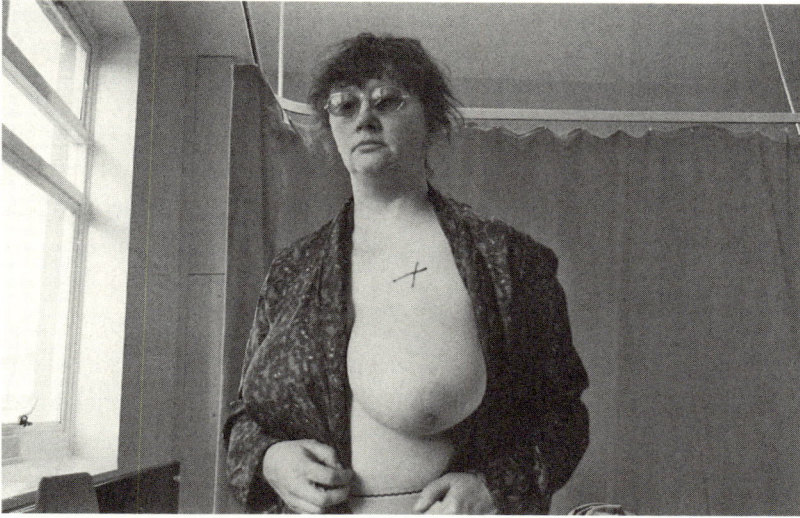

Figure 2. Jo Spence/Terry Dennett, *Marked Up for Amputation*. 1982. From The Cancer Project, Nottingham. (Courtesy of the Jo Spence Memorial Archive)

and critical, yet remaining attached to the emotional and frightening experiences I was undergoing" (*CS* 130).

The image not only instances the possibility of transcending the limitations of realistic documentation but actually draws force from the circumstances of its production. Terry Dennett, who stayed with Spence in the hospital when she was diagnosed, remarked of the photograph's scene of production, "Upset as we both were, we were aware that this time was a key one—the last day with two full breasts . . . [T]he actual image was not pre-scripted, it existed because in the morning a young doctor had walked up to [Spence's] bed and put the cross on her breast. So really this is a found image that was not post visualised."[12] For Dennett, the image stands out as "encapsulating the whole situation—the body as a target, the breast as a redundant object, Jo as a depersonalised medical subject."[13] Yet Spence herself, after she became ill, consistently rejected as too rigid and limiting any methodology or theory of representation that pretended to accurately present things as they are or to "encapsulate" the way they really happened. In a dialogue with Ross Coward in 1986, she pointed at the sustained gap between the kind of forensic endeavor she and Dennett explicitly sought and her self-reflexive awareness of the problematic inherent in the documentary mode. "At the same time as I am trying to work out how to take photographs of what is happening to me, I also know that whatever I am about to photograph isn't actually what is happening. That it is only the tip of the iceberg because of censorship and self-censorship, and because you can't show the structures which produce that situation" ("Body Talk?" qtd. in Evans, *Camerawork Essays* 1).

If the quest to represent the reality of illness was established as the missing link between a political (Marxist, feminist) consciousness and the desire to embody individual suffering, it was not a naive move but one highly aware of the limitations of self-representation. The crucial difference between Spence's cancer photographs and those that reflect her previous interest in women's cultural representation lies in the illness photographs' break from emphasizing the way social power relations construct cultural images and their new focus on the individual who is situated within and is subjugated by those cultural forces. Feeling "sick of medical people who viewed me as only an object of study or treatment . . . [and] equally sick of academics within my own field of discourse who wrote theories of the representation of bodies without in any way seeming to inhabit their own" (*CS* 130), Spence turned to her own lived experience of illness as a reference point that not only generated but continued to shape her creative endeavor. The photographs she made in the hospital ward provided her with "visual markers," and "act[ed] as touchstones for reliving memories and taking first faltering steps towards opening my mouth even wider to speak" (*CS* 131).

In the process of photographing herself later as an actor in scripted and staged tableaux, Spence continued to use these photographs, mnemonically, as a means of enforcing her final decision in 1982 to refuse mastectomy and radiotherapy and to have a simple lumpectomy followed by Gerson therapy and Chinese herbs. Her *Infantilization* series (figure 3) illustrates the kind of previsualised and pre-scripted work that evolved from these documentary photographs. Clearly, these staged tableaux make visible the patient's feelings of infantile regression and powerlessness, which the documentary mode failed to represent. Just as clearly, however, they have lost the indexical quality and reality effect of the hospital-ward

THE INVADING BODY

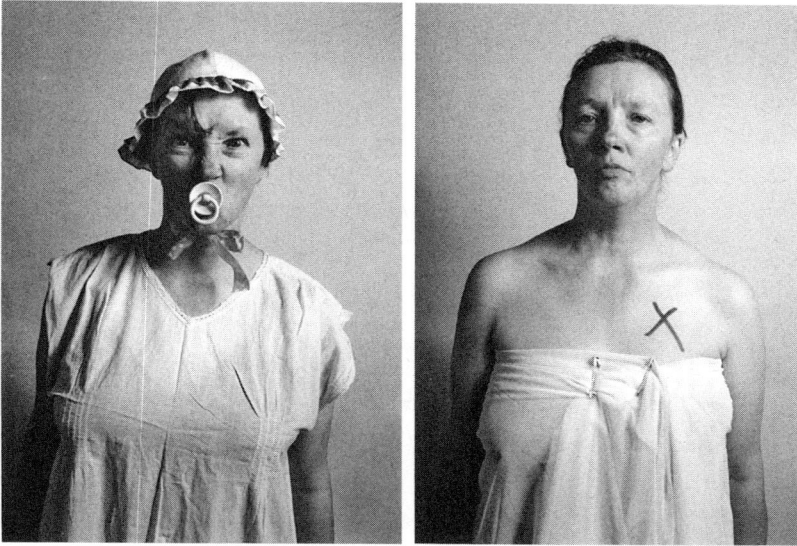

Figure 3. Jo Spence/Rosy Martin, *Infantilization*. 1984. From "The Picture of Health? Part 3." "Making visible the feelings of powerlessness and infantilization at the hands of the medical profession." (Courtesy of the Jo Spence Memorial Archive)

photographs. Although the process of their production is indebted to Spence's determination to rely on the documentary photographs indexically, as "touchstones," the props she selected as metaphors for the abject state of being "the 'naughty little daughter' . . . facing up to doctor/daddy and nurse/mummy" (*CS* 122),[14] insulate the feeling of infantile regression at the expense of the sense of fatal urgency imparted by the "marked up" self-portrait at the hospital.

The pacifier and baby cap and the safety pins holding a diaperlike sheet around the woman's chest—accompanied by the facial and body gestures of infantile rage—deflate and deplete the mark above the woman's breast. The dense symbolism that surrounds it turns the body mark from something that will instigate crucial consequences beyond the photograph's frame into just another prop in the sequence of symbolic devices. Overtly staged, these images remain cut off from the reality outside the photograph's frame—they personify an emotional state that is divorced from both the physical and the temporal (rather than the formally constituted) dimension of the experience of illness.

Yet to approach these images in isolation would be to disregard Spence's more complex treatment of the persistent demand of the sick body to be articulated. Her affirmation of an array of modes, or a gradient, for expressing what it means to be ill is manifest in her decision to present the *Infantilization* series side by side with both her hospitalization photographs and the photographs of the alternative treatment that she undertook after her discharge from the hospital. Compare the scripted tableaux to the picture *Alternative Health Treatment Using Traditional Chinese Medicine* (figure 4), which was not previsualized but taken as a mode of self-affirmation, documenting the alternative treatment Spence chose to adopt on declining the radical mastectomy and course of radiation prescribed by the orthodox medical establishment. However "real" this black and white photograph may seem, it is yet carefully constructed. Its subtle play of light and darker grays enhances the plastic quality of Spence's skin, making tangible every pore and line on her back and face. But it also works to naturalize the potentially alarming image of the four black incense needles that stick from her back. The shadows of the incense needles both resemble and blend with the shaded areas of Spence's shoulders and spine, and are repeated in the hollows of her cheek and temple. The smoke curling from the burning incense finds its formal parallel in the darker tufts of her uncombed hair. And yet, these clearly constructed visual parallels do not detract from the picture's reality effect, both in terms of its analogical function and in its ability to authenticate for the viewer the sense of the passing of time. The message the picture connotes of an harmonious relation between the sick artist and her chosen mode of treatment is inseparable from the particularity of the experience, which is poignantly denoted by the arrested rings of smoke, the frozen raised eyebrow, the corporeal, aging skin.

This denotative connection to the particularity of the photographed moment was consciously used by Spence as a means of reinforcing her sense of individual agency when her refusal to undergo traditional allopathic treatment for breast cancer raised an overwhelmingly general criticism. "I don't think I've ever been so lonely in my entire life," she said of that time; "[n]early everybody I knew thought I was mad" (*CS* 213).[15]

THE INVADING BODY

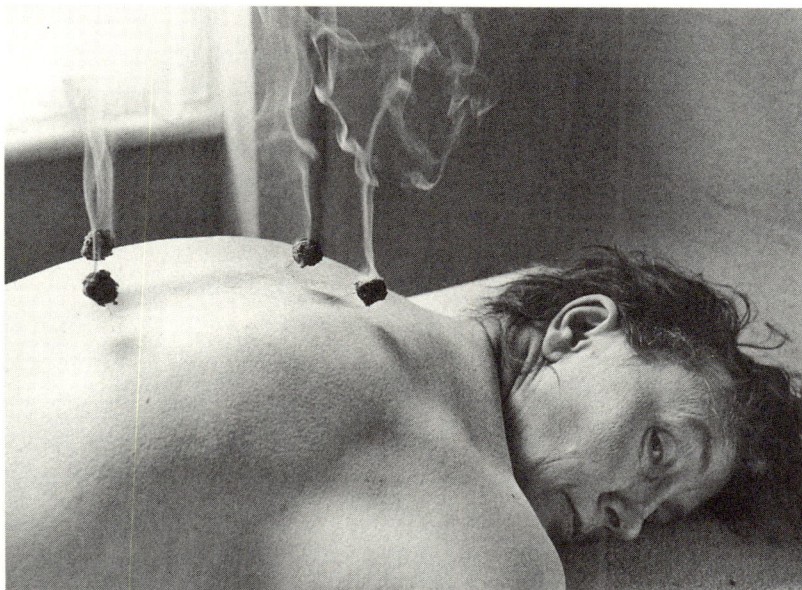

Figure 4. Maggie Murray, *Alternative Treatment Using Traditional Chinese Medicine.* 1984. From "The Picture of Health?" (Courtesy of the Jo Spence Memorial Archive)

True to her practice of obsessively documenting almost every aspect of her daily life, she asked a photographer friend, Maggie Murray,

> to take photographs of my alternative treatment as a confirmation that I had made the right choice. I could see from the photographs that I was clearly doing things to heal myself: juicing juices and mixing up herbs and doing exercise. In some way, these photographs were like my advocate's eye saying I needed to do these things to become well. I placed these images around me and looked at them a lot. I think I was beginning to learn to love myself. They gave me a lot of information about how gentle I was being with myself—a major shift from the steroids and antibiotics I had taken all my life as an asthmatic. (*CS* 213)

The photographs' literal message, "juicing juices and mixing up herbs," is inseparable from Spence's experiential and interpretive relation to them.

What she is shown as literally doing in the photographs is what enables her to receive them as a source of emotional and rational knowledge. The process of receiving the photographs, then, empowered her in the struggle with her illness in "real life." As a viewer, in addition to being the subject and object of her photographs, she could use their reality effect in a way that became instrumental to her process of healing.[16] Conversely, her continued engagement in the lived experience of treatment, and, at the same time, in the process of producing the healing images in which she played the roles of both object and subject, gradually shaped the double narrative of exhibition The Picture of Health? (1986). Her twofold ideological purpose there was, first, to launch a critique of "the cancer industry" by enlarging her hospitalization photographs and placing them next to her *Infantilization* series, and, second, to use her alternative treatment photographs to "make visible self-help methods of caring, as well as details on how to detoxify, physically and mentally" (*CS* 132).

Thus, in spite of the overt ideological thrust of the finished work—the "show" that came to be known as The Picture of Health?—to identify these photographs as ideological icons only would be too reductive and conceptually problematic. It would mean leaving out of the discussion the photographs' processes of production and reception, which, crucially, can account for their powerful "reality effect," the literal message that refers them to the actual struggle of the sick. Spence herself made a telling distinction between these cancer photographs and her earlier, explicitly ideological work with her naked body before her 1982 diagnosis.[17] Before she became ill she had photographed herself as a means of problematizing the culturally given representations of the female nude. "But that was totally different—the body I had put up on the wall then was not diseased and scarred. Those nudes had been about ideological things. Cancer was about my own history. So taking this step was profoundly difficult for me" (*CS* 213).[18] While I do not wish to deny the constructed, connotative meaning of the cancer photographs, as well as their potential political effect in increasing the audience's awareness of illness as a contested site of social relations of power, there is a persistent, personally urgent quality to them that stems directly from their denotative meaning—from

THE INVADING BODY

their power to enact the body's "demand in and for language" (Butler 67), poignantly experienced through the materiality of being sick.

The indexicality, or "reality effect," of Spence's cancer photographs should not be confused with a personal motive for the project or dismissed as a biographic detail external to the finished work. To do that would mean, once more, to separate the work from the dynamics of production and reception through which its reality effect is validated. Spence expected her audience to recognize and appreciate the same quality of contiguity with lived experience that had occasioned and actively sustained the production of these photographs—and was severely disappointed when viewers failed to respond to it. As she put it in her interview with Jan Zita Grover, recalling people's painful lack of response: "I thought, 'Don't you understand that I might be dying—that I've put up this work on the wall to help other people see that there are other ways to think about this illness?' And additionally, 'This isn't just an art work. This is an actual body that someone inhabits'" (*CS* 213–14). What she missed was a recognition of the lesson taught by illness—"how much," as she put it, "the body was not 'just a bloody sign' but something vulnerable that needed attention" (Stanley, *CS* 113).[19] And yet, the silence of the audience's reception is telling in itself. The audience's refusal to acknowledge the literal experience of illness demonstrates the culturally constructed prohibition on the gaze when it is confronted with the sick. Ironically, the very persistency of the literal message in these photographs, evident in their power to confront the viewers with the culturally repressed, both provokes and secures the audience's silence as a mark of resistance.

For Spence, the audience's lack of response was an extremely costly personal and professional crisis. It threw her, as she told Grover, into "the biggest minefield of silence I had ever been in my entire life . . . I had no way of knowing where I was going or what I was doing because nobody would speak to me" (*CS* 214). Eventually, however, her understanding of the dynamics of the audience's negative reception of the cancer photographs led her to address the system of values that dictates the cultural split between illness and health. In a 1987 proposal for a television program, which was taken up by BBC 2's Arena and broadcast two years later,

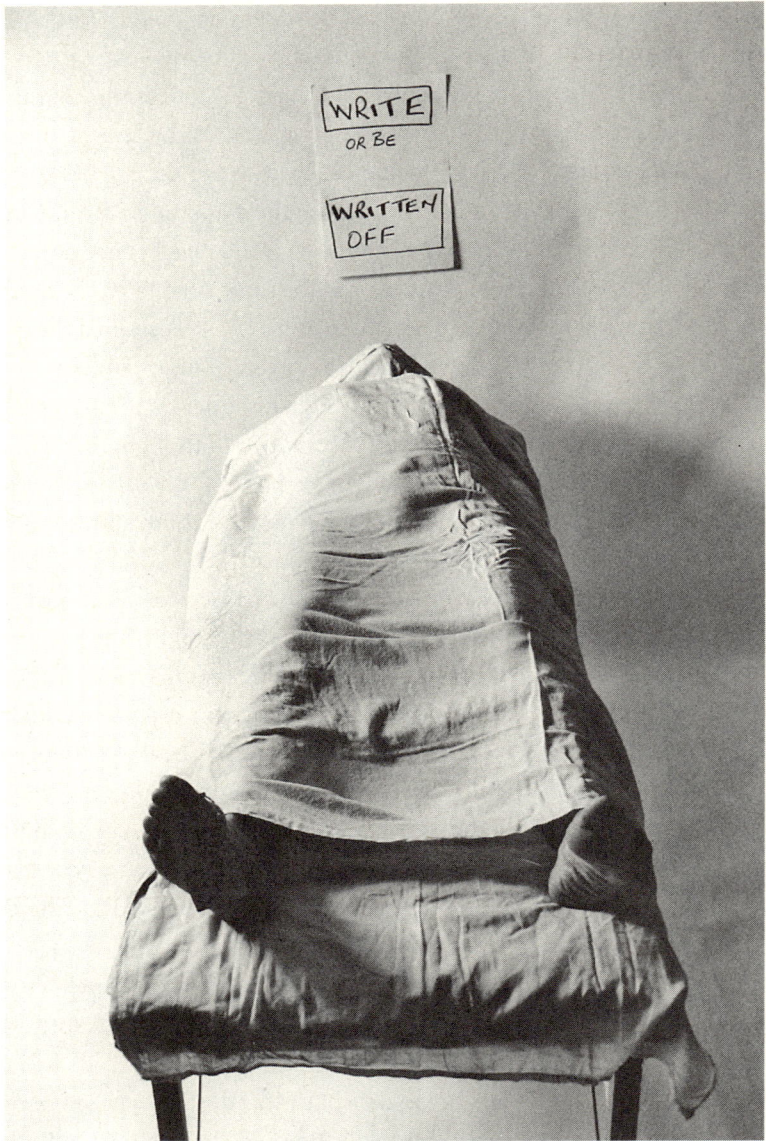

Figure 5. Jo Spence/David Roberts, *Write or Be Written Off*. 1988. "In 1983, after being diagnosed as having breast cancer, I silently faded away from the social and economic life of cultural production. At gallery openings instead of being asked 'How are you?' I was often asked 'What have you been doing?' Finally, it feels safe enough to speak to (or to endure the gaze of) only my husband, as I go into deep depression." (Courtesy of the Jo Spence Memorial Archive)

in 1989, she endeavored to deconstruct this institutionalized binary op-position through a dramatized examination of the pressure put on breast-cancer patients to wear a prosthesis after mastectomy. The pressure to hide "injuries, deformities, and amputations," even though such a conceal-ment "has no function other than a purely cosmetic one" (*CS* 125), was addressed by Spence as more than just an outward manifestation of the cultural repression of the sick: once imposed, she has argued, such acts of concealment carry a cultural life of their own inasmuch as they further re-pudiate the legitimacy of representing illness, in art as well as in daily life. In her proposal, Spence demands, first, to "consider what it means to be 'fit to be seen' . . . [to] look at the cosmetic value placed on health—how we are encouraged to be healthy in order to look good" (*CS* 126). And sec-ond, she wants to explore the ways in which "we conceal and hide images of ill-health from our lives" (*CS* 126). The proposal as a whole dramatizes her rejection of "ideas of health which see illness as the opposite of being well rather than part of a bodily continuum of health" (*CS* 126).

Her growing awareness of the cultural exclusion, and, thence, repres-sion, of visual signs of illness from the "bodily continuum of health" moved her back to her earlier engagement with the sick body as a sign, as something that might, indeed must, penetrate the audience's silence in order to be understood. As can be seen in figure 5 (*Write or Be Written Off*), the negative reception of the cancer photographs, while adding to the difficulties already imposed by illness, has nonetheless constructively influenced Spence's later work. This 1988 image retrospectively enacts Spence's feelings of loneliness and depression following the lack of re-sponse to her experience of illness—both on becoming physically ill and after her first exhibition of the cancer photographs. Clearly, the photo-graph also imparts the need to spell out—"write"—or otherwise discur-sively engage in what the audience can easily understand, which binds the individual's urge to express her idiosyncratic experience of illness with an awareness of the limitations imposed by culture on the processes of production and reception. With her body covered like a corpse in a morgue, it is only through the name written on her bare foot that a sense of individuality is momentarily implied. But then it is also immediately renounced, since, as the public has been taught by numerous movies and television shows, such a name tag is the very visual, cultural symbol of death or the state of being "written off."

Thus, the audience's silence in response to her cancer photographs gradually turned Spence away from the attempt to represent her individual experience and involved her, instead, in the politics of representation. During the second half of the 1980s she became focused on the political purpose of rearticulating signs of illness in a way that would render them more favorable to those who are most affected by them. At a time when, as she has said, "there was practically no one in this country to talk about cancer and the politics of cancer" (CS 216), she struggled not only to deconstruct visual signs and symbols of illness but also to reconstruct such signs "in ways which are more in the interests of those they signify than those who traditionally control signs' production and circulation" (CS 135).[20] "That's the lonely path I continued to walk until I collapsed with leukaemia" (CS 216), she said in the previously quoted interview with Jan Zita Grover in 1991, the last major interview she gave, a year before her death. This time around, aware that her illness was incurable, Spence again felt compelled to drastically revise her attitude toward the representation of illness.

The crisis of representation forced by leukemia branched out in two major and irreconcilable directions, both crucially related to Spence's awareness of leukemia as a terminal illness. On the one hand, she renounced her political engagement and turned inward to the kind of identity search and self-care already suggested in her alternative treatment course; on the other hand, she was compelled to reevaluate her long-held concept of selfhood as continually evolving and to come to terms with the idea of extinction, of the death of the self. The difference between her relation to the experience of breast cancer and to the experience of leukemia is most immediately shown in her decision to quit the political struggle and to concentrate on what was happening to herself. "This time around," she told Jan Zita Grover, "I'm spending my time trying to decide what story my illness is telling Me rather than trying to impose a narrative onto other people that I still don't even understand myself. That was what I did with breast cancer, as I now see it" (CS 216). This shift from a political model of photography to photography as a mode of understanding the

THE INVADING BODY

self was influenced in part by her years of engagement in phototherapy, which she developed alongside her work on the politics of cancer. And yet, it was the undeniable seriousness of her physical condition that shattered her trust in the usefulness of the political model: "I then [in 1982] thought immediately about how to be useful—how to turn my illness into something useful [for others]. I think to some extent I abused myself: I was so anxious to be useful that I exploited myself in some ways" (CS 212). By contrast, she realizes in 1991 that "choosing to go like an Amazon into the lion's den over and over again in order to be politically useful is just too energy-consuming and too conflictual. In the end it didn't seem to me to serve any function at all, so it feels at this point as if I will never do anything again except look after myself" (CS 217).

The constant, time-consuming care required in "looking after myself with leukaemia"—which Spence has compared to "having a newborn baby to look after" (CS 217)—is one obvious aspect of daily life with the disease that rendered uncertain the possibility of her working in the future. Yet even at this point of unrelenting physical challenge, her usual method of "shooting first and asking questions afterwards" (Dennett, "PhotoTherapy" n.pag.) endured. She has, in fact, maintained her career-long habit of conducting a visual diary: "I take my snapshots," she told Grover; "I've been keeping a visual diary about the crisis of representation that I'm passing through. I will probably write about it one day" (CS 217). Thus, her "crisis of representation" stemmed not so much from her physical disability, from an inability to "shoot" the pictures, but was, rather, the result of a cognitive impasse that made her habit of "asking questions afterwards" excruciatingly difficult. Her inability to select and construct her visual diary in a meaningful way, as she used to do in the past, testifies to the psychic collapse she was undergoing, which was augmented by her research into the clinical aspects of leukemia. Spence was aware that her present condition "was potentially far more debilitating than the breast cancer she had managed to stabilize naturopathically for eight years" (CS 222).[21] But at the same time that she realized the futility of the political, utilitarian model, she was also forced to relinquish basic assumptions about the self that had emerged from and were in turn reinforced by her previous endeavors to represent the experience of illness.

Her assumption about self-care and its promise for individual growth, for example, which had led to and been dramatized in her engagement in phototherapy, no longer proved relevant to the representation of an experience of illness for which there was no cure. Likewise, her concept of the self as a process, which had sustained her autobiographical photographs in both their political and their therapeutic expressions, failed to meet the sense of ultimate disintegration and of imminent death with which she was forced to grapple. Before she became ill with leukemia, Spence conceived of and strove to represent the self as an ever-evolving, nonessentialist entity equally shaped by societal pressures and the individual's endeavor to challenge those pressures by identifying and (re)defining her place within them. As she has put it in her autobiography, "there is no peeling away of layers to reveal a 'real' self, just a constant reworking process. I realize that I am a process" (*Putting Myself in the Picture* 86). Notwithstanding her nonessentialist vocabulary, however, it is precisely the underlying sense of agency, of some part of the self that is watchful and can testify to herself as "a process," that itself became liable to change as a result of the experience of terminal illness. Furthermore, it was the desire to regain her collapsed sense of agency—to hold on to the degree of control afforded by her method of self-documentation—that helped Spence to overcome her creative paralysis. Eventually, she began to outline the last autobiographical project she was involved in before her death, which she named The Final Project.

The Final Project was never completed. The original plan included two major elements: "an ongoing photo documentation with David Roberts of her health and survival treatments, and, dependent on her energy levels, photo theatre and photo-therapy sessions [in collaboration with Terry Dennett] around areas connected with death and death culture, backed up by a study of approaches to death in different cultures" (*CS* 222).[22] However, as her health declined rapidly, Spence had to reconcile herself to the fact that she would never again engage directly in photography. "[O]ut of frustration and necessity" (Dennett, "Notes on 'The Final Project'" n.pag.), she decided instead "to use the existing material from her archive to create the kind of pictures she would have taken" (*CS* 222), re-

THE INVADING BODY

turning to techniques she had already used in the 1970s of projecting images onto photographs and sandwiching slides together.

Metamorphosis (figure 6) is the only image, or rather a sequence of images, that the project yielded. According to Terry Dennett, who produced the work after Spence's death according to her specific instructions, this image was intended to be one of a number of pre-planned and scripted "super-impositions" that represented "substitute selves"—a set of allegorical images that featured Spence predominantly as a doll, a skeleton, and, finally, a mask ("Notes on 'The Final Project'" n.pag.). Although the project was not sufficiently advanced to establish how these elements would have been interwoven, Spence prescribed the treatment of individual images and bequeathed to Dennett the legacy of selecting and producing at least one photograph after her death. "As her collaborator," says Dennett, "I was entrusted with the task of taking a photograph which 'should not be too gruesome a death or near death portrait' and then finish it in accordance with her wishes for presentation in a suitable context when she had gone" ("Metamorphosis" n.pag.). This kind of joint work was not exceptional in Spence's and Dennett's long history of photographic coproduction (many of the breast-cancer photographs followed the same line of collaboration). If anything, Dennett was extra-careful, this time, to implement Spence's ideas as accurately as possible, conscientiously comparing his role to that of a legal executor.[23]

Metamorphosis consists of four consecutive images produced by the sandwiched slide technique. The basic image is that of Spence's head, taken shortly after her death and frozen as if in sleep. The head has been doubled (top two images) and then condensed, so that the two heads gradually crush into one another until they lose their facial features and, in the last image (bottom image), strikingly come to resemble a woman's sexual organ. Spence had meticulously previsualized and scripted both the sandwiching technique and the allegorical structure of rebirth implied by the metamorphosis of self-division (the double head) and its reemergence as the organ of fertility and symbol of connection in the world.

In the context of Spence's oeuvre, what is striking about *Metamorphosis* is neither its allegorical representation of seasonal regeneration nor the

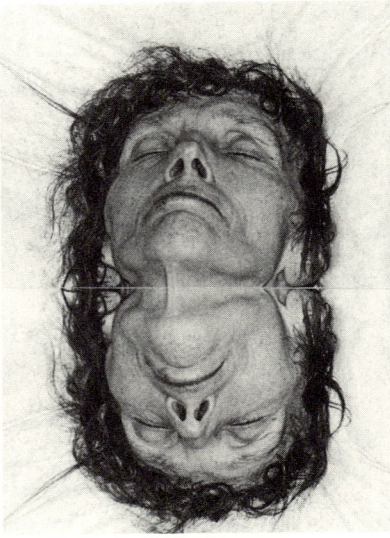
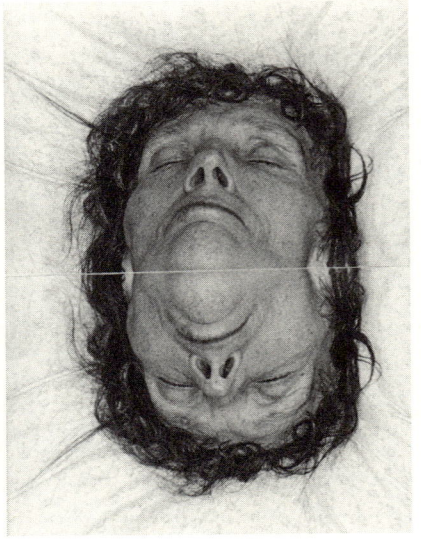
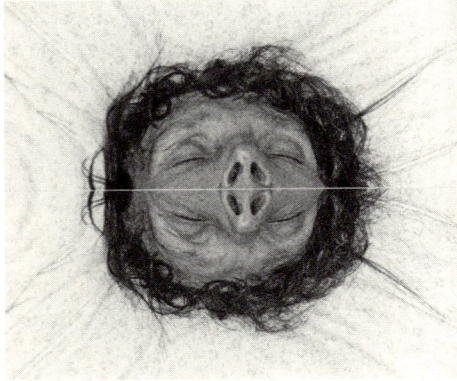
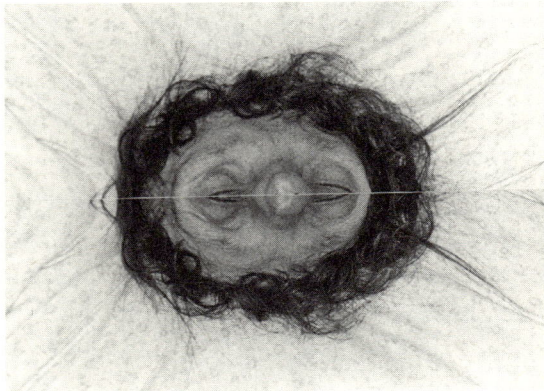

explicit configuration of such "taboo" subjects as sex and death. The allegorical approach to death in *Metamorphosis* clearly aligns it with the large body of illness narratives that achieve a mythic formulation of the experience of terminal illness. In her seminal study of mythic paradigms in illness narratives, discussed earlier in this book, Ann Hunsaker Hawkins comments on

the extent to which these very personal accounts of illness, though highly individualized, tend to be confined to certain repeated themes— themes of an archetypal, mythic nature. Over and over again, the same metaphorical paradigms are repeated in pathographies: the paradigm of regeneration, the idea of illness as battle, the athletic ideal, the journey into a distant country, and the mythos of healthy-mindedness. (27).

Indeed, what stands out in this photograph is not the depiction of "universal" themes but rather the total absence of reference to Spence's idiosyncratic experience of dying. This absence, in turn, attracts attention to the photograph's double resistance: first, to the practice of self-documentation as a mode of representing individual experience, and, second, to the idea of photography as a medium that can analogically refer to the "real," prephotographed reality.

That the basic image—the head in figure 6a—complies with Spence's own wishes is evident from her instruction, quoted previously, to choose for this scripted project a photograph that "should not be too gruesome a death or near death portrait." Accordingly, the woman's face in the "base" image shows no sign of illness or of imminent death. Devoid of a body and of any other mark of lived experience, its expression of anguish is contextualized, rather, by the allegory of rebirth, which the sequence as a whole sustains. At the level of photographic treatment, moreover, the

Figure 6. Jo Spence/Terry Dennett, *Metamorphosis.* 1991–92. From The Final Project (unfinished). Recognizing that she was about to die, Spence discussed with Dennett how she wanted her death to be depicted. A photograph of her taken shortly after she died has been manipulated to describe a return to the womb, a dramatic and moving disappearance. (Courtesy of the Jo Spence Memorial Archive)

work's allegorical orientation and its underlying aim of opposing a naive view of photography as a record of the real are congruent with Spence's prescription of the projected and sandwiched slide techniques that monitor the sequence of images. These techniques serve to undermine the belief in photography as a mode that can capture "the real" inasmuch as they highlight photography's deceptive qualities. As Dennett has put it in the text that accompanied the presentation of the work in 1995, *Metamorphosis* intends to expose the idea of photographic realism as "a lie, for on closer examination the images are seen to be constructed from a single photograph" ("Metamorphosis" n. pag.).

And yet, it is hard to reconcile this twofold resistance, both to illness self-documentation and to photographic documentation at large, with the original outline of The Final Project, in which self-documentation was conceived of as having a substantial part. Moreover, Spence's career-long practice of conducting a visual diary, which she pursued until the last months of her life, is incompatible with such a resistance since it enacts her very trust in the value of documenting individual lived experience.

Two major reasons are given by Dennett, in different contexts, to account for The Final Project's deviation from the original plan: Spence's physical inability to take her own pictures and her anxiety that her declining physical appearance would no longer serve either her therapeutic or her political purposes. "*Metamorphosis*," says Dennett, "was conceived at a time when the leukaemia which eventually killed [Spence] had already made it difficult for her to sustain the energy to take her own pictures and when she was finally forced to seriously think about the possibilities of her death" ("Metamorphosis," n.pag.). However, since Spence was surrounded and cared for by her husband and friends—all professional photographers with whom she had often collaborated in creating her autobiographical work in the past—the fact that she was too ill to take her own pictures should not have prevented her from documenting the last stages of illness had she so desired. Far more telling is the second motive given by Dennett for the change in the original plan, that is, for the conscious omission from the project of the kind of reality effect Spence had never hesitated to produce in her autobiographical representation of breast cancer.

THE INVADING BODY

As Jo Spence's illness progressed, her physical appearance deterio-
rated to a point where she felt that direct photography of her body
could no longer give images that correspond with her therapeutic
aims or her mental impression of herself as an active cancer patient—
"mind self" and "mirror self" became so rapidly divergent that she
could no longer identify with the ill looking stranger she saw in her
mirror each morning.

Given her visual appearance she contended that a documentary approach was therefore only likely to identify her as a victim rather than
the fighter she was attempting to be. As a long time critic of "victim
photography" she therefore decided to adopt an indirect allegorical
approach to the project by creating a series of substitute selves. ("Notes
on 'The Final Project,'" n.pag.)

An occupation with the personal and the "therapeutic," then, has replaced
the overtly political double narrative observed in her breast-cancer photographs, that of resisting orthodox medicine and of offering an alternative mode of care. Still, The Final Project relies on Spence's former view
of the self as evolving and reworked vis-à-vis social pressures: the photographs are perceived to be successful inasmuch as they reinforce her self-
image as a "fighter" and fail if they represent her as "a victim" of cancer.

The decision to relinquish the documentary mode when it no longer
yields an empowering effect is, thus, compatible with Spence's earlier assertion that the self is constructed through and through. If there is no inherent core to the self, self-representation may well be evaluated by its enabling or disabling effect. Yet, what is striking about Dennett's account is
the immediate connection Spence has drawn between her "mirror-self"
and documentary photography insofar as the "direct photography of her
body" is conceived to be just as misleading and false as "the ill looking
stranger she saw in her mirror each morning." Such a direct placement of
self-documentation and of "mirror-self" on the same plane in terms of
their identical effect discloses a residual conviction in the denotative
qualities of photography that, no matter how false to one's "mind-self,"
carry the same visual, evidential truth as in one's encounter with her reflection in the mirror. This implicit acknowledgment of the evidential

force of the documentary mode suggests Spence's sense that one's visual appearance as recorded by photography carries a spectatorial truth so powerful that it must be consciously resisted and countered by such "indirect" rhetorical strategies of allegory and symbol as have been employed in *Metamorphosis.*

Spence's refusal to deal directly with the body is uncannily similar to her own audience's resistance to her embodied, sick self in the breast-cancer photographs. By opting for an allegorical approach to death, by evading, that is, the uncontrollable physical aspects of terminal illness through the creation of a series of "substitute selves," The Final Project strangely reiterates the audience's silence/repression in response to The Cancer Project. Figure 7 (*Untitled*), the only published photograph in the self-documentary mode that was taken shortly before Spence's death, further enhances the sense of the denial of the reality of dying. It shows Spence on a "good day," emaciated but smiling and in perfect control, "photographing visitors to her room at the Marie Curie Hospice, Hampstead" (*CS* 227).[24] It therefore discloses Spence's willingness to use self-documentation, the "direct photography of her body," only when the medium's evidential force proves to be enabling. This is clearly the portrait of "an active cancer patient," "a fighter," rendered visually in command not only of the entrance—and visitors—to her room but also of the way she will be viewed by others after her death.

Understandable as the wish for self-control surely is, Spence's resistance of documentary photography when its literal message fails to be empowering, and particularly when it serves to produce a "gruesome death or near death portrait," jars with her early claims that "the camera is not a window on the world, nor are meanings of pictures fixed, but . . . visual signs (in this case photographs) are in themselves sites of struggle" (*Putting Myself in the Picture* 119). Her refusal to produce "direct" images of physical deterioration betrays, rather, her awareness of the persistence of the literal message in documentary photography. It is through her refusal to expose the uncontrollable particularities of terminal illness that a sense of Roland Barthes' "photographic paradox"[25] is inadvertently evoked in its capacity not only to connote but also to denote, at

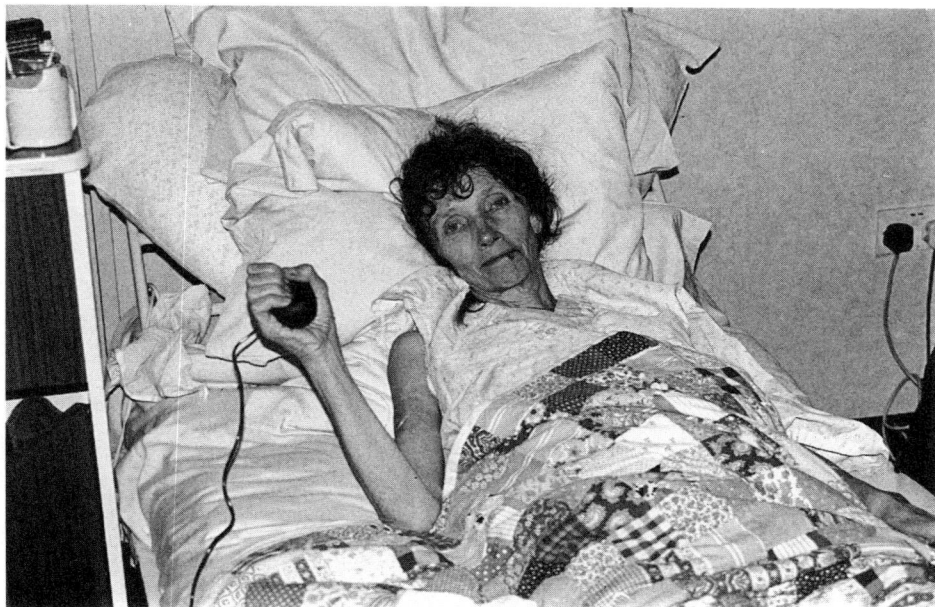

Figure 7. Terry Dennett, *Untitled*. 1992. Jo Spence on a "good day" shortly before her death, photographing visitors to her room at the Marie Curie Hospice, Hampstead. (Courtesy of the Jo Spence Memorial Archive)

once to construct and to directly refer to the reality beyond the photograph's given frame.

Victor Burgin's idea of the audience's active role in constructing photographic significance may help to further illuminate this point. In the introduction to her *Family Frames: Photography, Narrative, and Postmemory,* Marianne Hirsch usefully interprets Burgin's formulation of the relationship between photographers and their audience in terms of their mutual production of "a screen" of ideology and dominant mythologies that actively shape photographic representation. Burgin, says Hirsch,

suggests that "the structure of representation—point-of-view and frame—is intimately implicated in the reproduction of ideology (the 'frame of mind' of our 'points-of-view')." But the structure of looking is reciprocal: photographer and viewer collaborate on the reproduction of ideology. Between the viewer and the recorded object, the viewer encounters, and/or projects, a screen made up of dominant mythologies and preconceptions that shapes the representation. (Burgin 146, qtd in Hirsch 7)

Burgin's insights on photography are highly pertinent to a discussion of Spence's work. Spence had in fact studied with Burgin at the Polytechnic of Central London (now the University of Westminster) and tried to apply Burgin's critical theory to her work on breast cancer. In particular, as she put it, she wanted "to foreground some of the structured and structuring absences and silences which dominate forms of representation" (*CS* 129).[26] Yet, what stands out in the final, allegorical approach to death are Spence's own "structured and structuring" absence and silence on the issue of her impending death. Furthermore, her desire to control all aspects of the image and, thus, to dictate the way she will be seen (as a fighter, an active patient, and so on) results in the negation of the viewer's role in the reciprocal engagement of the photographer and her audience with the recorded object—that is, with terminal illness and imminent death.

Possibly, as Evans has suggested, *Metamorphosis* is Spence's "attempt to make her mark on imminent death, on the event that is most uncontrollable of all"; the cyclic allegory is, thus, an endeavor to "make death meaningful and thus restore to it a sense of its being part of a life" (Evans 258). However, what is interesting about *Metamorphosis* is just that it is robbed of a life, or of idiosyncratic experience. Schematic and nonindividualized, it is rather a representation of Life than of a life. Perhaps, then, as Evans alternately suggests, Spence was pointing here "to the inadequacy in the end of metaphors of 'control' which are based on a fantasy prevalent in much of our culture—that death can be made good, that we can get something positive out of it, and so avoid the terror, anger and confusion that death evokes" (258). But such a preoccupation with the futility of cultural images of control is undercut both by Spence's refusal to acknowledge and confront her physical loss of control, evident in her rejected "mirror-image"; and by the telling lack of any indication to the contingent and inevitably idiosyncratic emotional processing of the experience of facing death.

THE INVADING BODY

While apparently pursuing Spence's resistance to the so-called realistic tradition in photography, *Metamorphosis* remains alienated from her personal reality of "terror, anger and confusion" in a way that the breast-cancer tableaux were not. The most significant difference between The Final Project and the rest of Spence's illness photographs is the disappearance or silencing of the subject's/photographer's individual experience of illness. This erasure or repression of her experience of dying is hardly a return to the consciously critical, "external" political perspective of the hospital-ward photographs. As we have seen, the photographic development of Spence's relation to her illness since the hospital-ward pictures were made emphasizes, rather, her process of learning to include her subjectivity and lived experience within the representation of illness as a crucial element of her photographs' testimonial force. Placed in the context of her oeuvre, Spence's final decision, in *Metamorphosis,* to exclude the experience of dying persistently suggests her awareness of the visual power of the photographic literal message.

Granted, Spence's methodology and thought had striven to question traditional documentary practices, and to align photography with theater and other performance arts, years before photography theory almost unanimously celebrated photographs as constructed visual sites of struggle. And yet, as this chapter has shown, the production and reception processes of her illness photographs acknowledge the evidential force of photography, however tacitly and even reluctantly. The tension between the contiguous and the constructed elements in her autobiographical work on illness is not unique to The Final Project—it is only revealed here more forcefully than before through the mechanism of repression. All of her illness photographs—the "realistic" hospital-ward photographs, the scripted tableaux, and, finally, the unfinished self-allegories—constitute a gradient of more or less accentuated tension between the indexically contingent and the previsualized and planned. If The Final Project demonstrates a positive thematic break from previous concerns with self-representation as well as from an explicitly political purpose, in terms of its metaphotographic undercurrent, the reflection on the relation between the documentary practice and reality "out there," it comes to reiterate—albeit by repudiation—Spence's career-long preoccupation with the photographic paradox. The explanatory power of Barthes' photographic paradox and its significance to autobiographical illness photographs will be discussed in the concluding section of the next chapter, where I place illness photographs within the current theoretical inquiry into the controversial relation of word and image, or the interfaces of narrated and spatial compositions. But first, to test my view of a gradient of tensed relations between indexical and symbolic elements in autobiographical illness photographs, I will turn to examine Hannah Wilke's different emphasis on the audience's role in establishing and resisting the truth-value of her cancer photographs.

5

HANNAH WILKE: PERFORMING GRIEF

JO SPENCE'S FINAL PROJECT IS INADVERTENTLY STRUCTURED
by the absence of the sick body and the photographer's anxiety about self-
control. By contrast, Hannah Wilke's series of photographs of terminal
illness, *Intra-Venus,* consciously foregrounds the risk of self-exposure
through direct photographs of her sick body. This is not just a different
selection of subject matter and photographic treatment but an open, and
far more risky, approach to her audience. Rather than try to control (or
close off) the "screen of expectations" that circumscribe and determine
what the audience will see, Wilke allows her viewers to participate in
shaping her representation of critical illness. One of the crucial consequences of this decision is that even as she attempts to anticipate and ma-
neuver the audience's reaction, she also risks manipulation by the audience. As we shall see, the audience's collaborative construction of the
"screen" of projected visual expectations that surrounds the recorded object may result in reproducing the cultural and visual clichés about the
terminally ill that her work has set out to resist.

Such risky combination of self-exposure and openness to diverse, and
at times antagonistic, interpretations has informed the reception of Wilke's
photography and body performance since the 1970s. Her self-portrait
photographs of the 1970s and 1980s, for example, were critiqued by fem-

inists for their narcissistic self-display. As Amelia Jones has said, her work was disparaged as ideologically equivocal, since by "objectifying herself in the photographs as she does, in assuming the conventions associated with a stripper," the work was seen "to end up by reinforcing what it intended to subvert" (Hess 93, qtd. in Jones 4). Figure 8, a detail of Wilke's Super-t-art 1974 exhibition, is an illustration of the work that Lucy Lippard has condemned as "seductive," "confusing the roles of beautiful woman and artist, flirt and feminist" (125, 126, qtd. in Jones 5). Jones's own argument is that the structure of narcissism enables Wilke to empower the position of a woman in patriarchy because "it confuses the conventional separation between the woman as object and subject of making that devalues women by consigning them to remain in the former role" (6). Thus, "narcissism instantiates the radical unknowability of the subject in representation and thwarts the oppositional logic by which women are consigned to a negative pole of 'immanence,' per Beauvoir, or (non)being within western thought" (Jones 7).

The same argument in favor of "radical narcissism" and its promise of social and psychological change underlies Jones's view of Wilke's 1992 *Intra-Venus* photographs and seems to have been resurrected in Jo Anna Isaak's recent celebration of Wilke's (and Spence's) illness photographs as enacting women's particular use of primary narcissism's "relation to laughter and laughter's indissoluble relation to revolution and freedom" (54). Yet, to view Wilke's last project, which documents her experience of lymphoma before her death in 1993, either as "forc[ing] the viewer to confront his or her expectations about the appearance of the female body in visual representations" (Jones 9), or as "the clearest example we are likely to get" of Freud's notion of "the triumph of narcissism" described in terms of the ego's ability to utilize the "traumas of the external world . . . [as] occasions for it to gain pleasure" (Isaak 50), is to subordinate Wilke's idiosyncratic experience of illness to a more inclusive feminist endeavor to subvert traditional representations and to revisualize the female body. To my mind, identifying these photographs as either feminist or narcissistic is both reductive and conceptually problematic. Apart from the potential audience of exclusively feminist and psychoanalytically oriented viewers, Wilke's disclosures of disease and the effects of treatment address

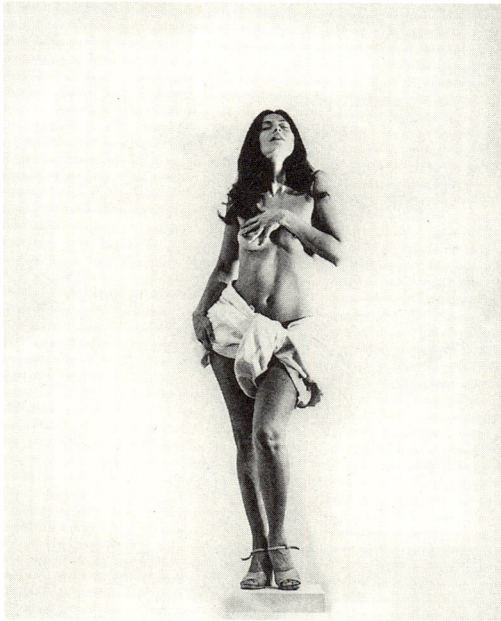

Figure 8. Hannah Wilke, Detail of *Hannah Wilke Super-T-Art.* Performalist Self-Portrait with Christopher Geircke. 1974. (Photo by D. James Dee. One of 20 photographs mounted on board, 40 x 32 inches each. Copyright 2005 Marsie, Emanuelle, Damon, and Andrew Scharlatt. Courtesy Ronald Feldman Fine Arts, New York.)

a heterogeneous actual audience as well as the wide range of culturally dominant beliefs, expectations, and fears that separate cancer imaginatively and morally from other types of sickness. Clearly, moreover, the photographs impose further divisions on the self-alienating structure of narcissism by representing a subject who examines her own process of physical transformation and deterioration, where the body is not externalized, projected, or passively contained like a mirror image—or subjected to the photographer's feminist or other ideological agenda—but actively takes over, undergoing uncontrollable and unwanted changes. On close inspection, the thematic continuity both Jones and Isaak note between Wilke's illness photographs and her whole oeuvre becomes crucially problematized.

Thus, only apparently does figure 9 repeat figure 8's statuesque self-assurance and self-containment. The self-confidence suggested by the

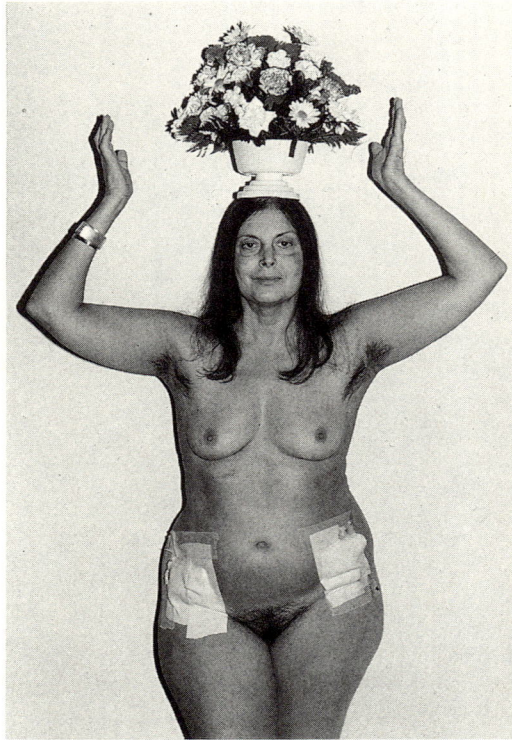

Figure 9. Hannah Wilke, *Intra-Venus Series No. 1*. 1991–92. January 30, 1992. (One of 2 panels. Chromagenic supergloss prints, 71½ x 47½ inches each. Photo by Dennis Cowley. Courtesy Ronald Feldman Fine Arts, New York.)

steady gaze, smiling face, and the act of balancing of a bowl of flowers is compositionally subverted through the white triangle of bowl and two hospital pads, blood-stained and implying the fragility of the cancerous body on which the head and flowers stand. The stained pads at once participate in tracing the contours of the body through the white triangle that echoes Wilke's head and hips and at the same time resist the image's aesthetic arrangement by introducing a contingent element alien to its formal composition: the vulnerable, oozing, wounded body, whose presence does not need to be explicitly shown here but is persistently evoked by the covering bandages. By pointing indexically to Wilke's prephotographic reality, the stained pads and the sick body they metonymically invoke paradoxically both validate and subvert the possibility of a citation

THE INVADING BODY

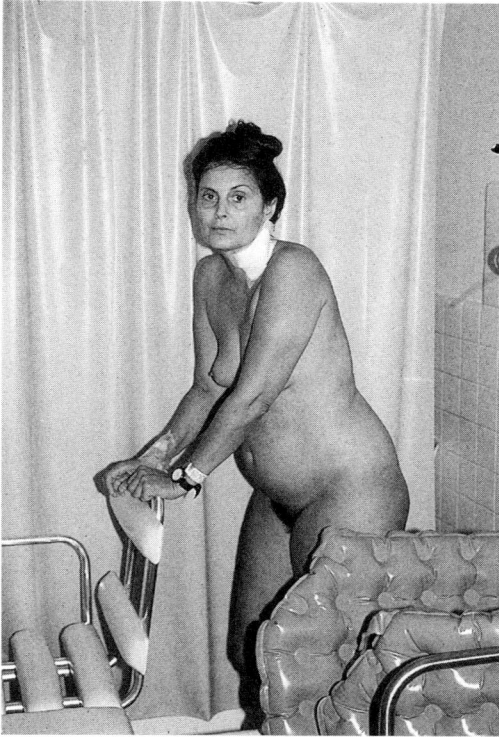

Figure 10. Hannah Wilke, *Intra-Venus Series No. 9*. 1991–92. October 26, 1991. (71½ x 47½ inches. Photo by Donald Goddard. Courtesy Ronald Feldman Fine Arts, New York.)

from her own earlier work. While iconically invoking Wilke's saintlike pose in figure 8, the qualitative difference in the level of exposure in the two images recapitulates the gap between Wilke's "narcissistic feminist" self-portraits of the 1970s and 1980s and her later preoccupation with bodily collapse. The illness photographs do not wholly reject, but significantly complicate the early tension between the artist's subjectivity and her assumed role as an object. In drawing attention to the continuous, literal elements that identify the recorded object with the subject outside the frame, Wilke has modified the sharp duality of subject and object, and has rearticulated this duality in terms of a continuum of interdependent subject-object positions.

Granted, as Jones and Isaak also contend, Wilke's play with cultural

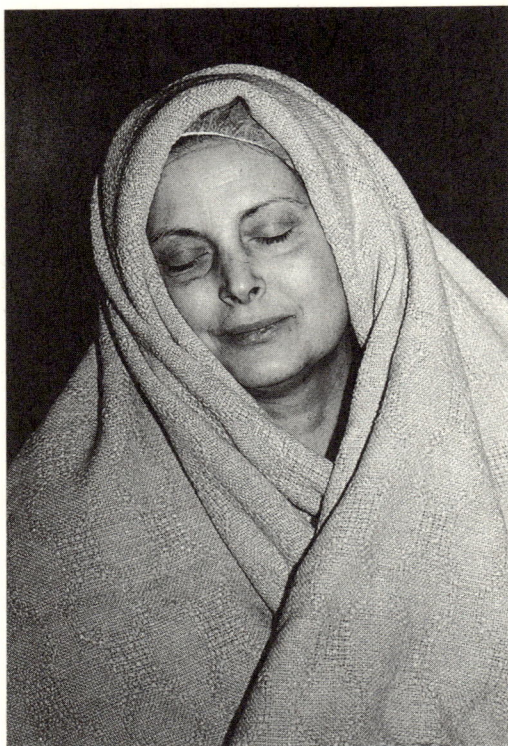

Figure 11. Hannah Wilke, *Intra-Venus Series No. 4*. 1991–92. February 19, 1992. (One of 2 panels. Chromagenic supergloss prints, 71½ x 47½ inches each. Photo by Dennis Cowley. Courtesy Ronald Feldman Fine Arts, New York.)

references and conventional poses invests the utterly personal reality of her imminent death with borrowed, shared cultural identities and values. But these cultural messages are always counterbalanced by the contiguous particularity of the photographs' indexical elements. In the middle of a hospital room she poses as a playboy bunny, her neck bandaged and her lush nakedness warm against the rigidity of hospital furniture (figure 10). The pastel pink and blue colors of the traditional "doll" shine hard on the cold plastic surfaces of curtain, chair and cushions, accenting the shared metonymy of anonymous dispensability that ironically unites sex objects and terminal patients. Simultaneously, they palely echo the red and blue colors traditionally associated with the Virgin Mary, a recurring association that other photographs foreground. Metonymy turned metaphor

THE INVADING BODY

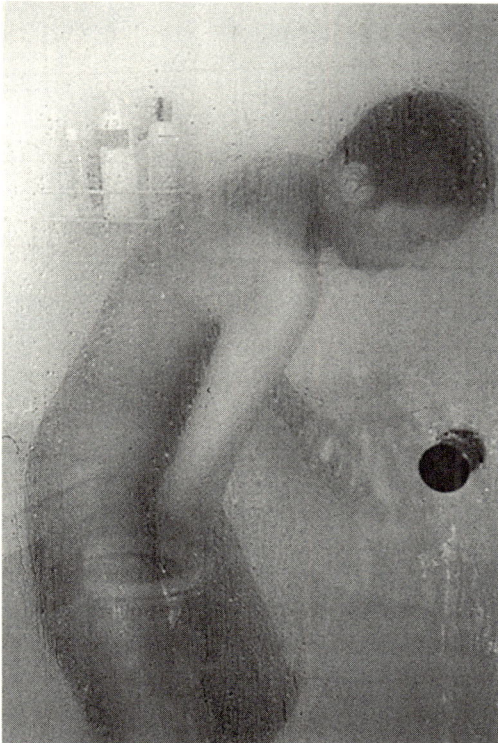

Figure 12. Hannah Wilke, *Intra-Venus Series No. 12.* 1991–92. December 15, 1992. (71½ x 47½ inches. Photo by Donald Goddard. Courtesy Ronald Feldman Fine Arts, New York.)

seems to be Wilke's preferred rhetorical figure. In a series of five photographs titled *Brushstrokes,* the effects of chemotherapy are represented through lessening loose wads of hair, which, as Jones has said, "are signifiers not only of Wilke's cancer but of the Holocaust that claimed millions of Jews during World War II" (12). In her most famous photograph (figure 11) her bald head is wrapped with a blue hospital blanket, infusing the metonymy of sickness with the borrowed emblem of Christian sainthood. Another photograph, taken, significantly, during a period of remission, shows her washing in the shower, where, like the heroine of Hitchcock's *Psycho,* she seems equally unaware of the camera and the lurking murderer (figure 12). In these and other photographs, the complexity of Wilke's culturally assimilated "self" is highlighted and informed

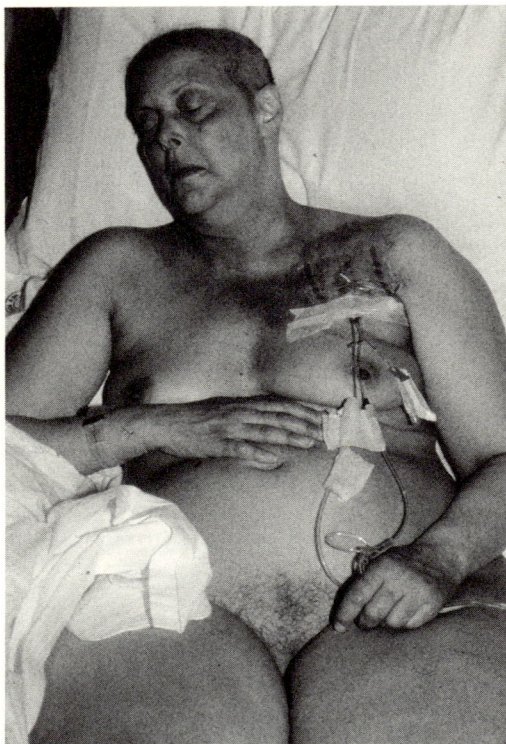

Figure 13. Hannah Wilke, *Intra-Venus Series No. 3.* 1991–92. August 17, 1992. (One of 3 panels. Chromagenic supergloss prints, 71½ x 47½ inches each. Courtesy Ronald Feldman Fine Arts, New York.)

by her position as a critically sick woman, an artist, and a subject aware of her self-fashioning by maps of visual signifiers.

Yet, this accumulative vision of a culturally saturated, embodied, and gendered self does far more than simply display "the whole repertoire of poses available to women, including the last—the grotesque, dying crone" (Isaak 50). As a whole, it rather accentuates the constant tension between Wilke's performance of conventional icons and the metonymic invocations of her lived experience of illness. The crucial distinction between cultural citation and lived experience culminates in the extremely disturbing chemotherapy photographs. Wilke's playful mastery over cultural and rhetorical codes pales in comparison with the exposure of the self she allows in the chemotherapy photographs precisely because these are

THE INVADING BODY

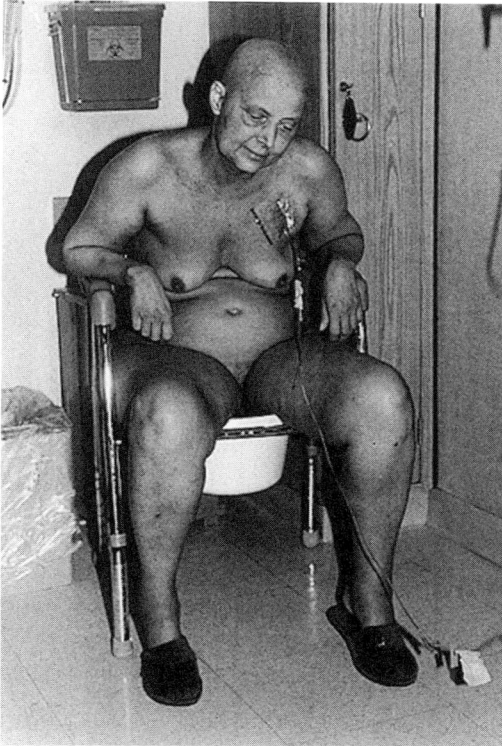

Figure 14. Hannah Wilke, *Intra-Venus Series No. 10*. 1991–92. June 22, 1992. (71½ x 47½ inches. Photo by Donald Goddard. Courtesy Ronald Feldman Fine Arts, New York.)

not "poses," let alone "poses available to women," but indexes of real endurance and suffering that cannot be shed. The bare messages of pain and sadness in those photographs (figures 13 and 14) signal no triumph over "the traumas of the external world"; they can be understood only through the evident traumas of the lived, embodied self. This does not mean, however, that the photographs are isolated records of Wilke's experience in the sense that they fail to engage in cultural work. Besides forming an unequivocal reminder of mortality, these photographs do significant ethical work in shocking the audience into a recognition of moral and rhetorical complicity. By engaging the taboo of cancer, they force the viewers to confront their own acceptance and perpetuation of the imagery of agony, disgust, guilt, and shame that saturates cancer in our society. The physical marks of illness are Wilke's, but the moral blemish involves the audience. Through their stark, utterly personal self-disclosure, the photographs resist the culturally ingrained myth of cancer as "a mindless It," "the disease of the Other [proceeding by] an invasion of 'alien' or 'mutant' cells" (Sontag, *Illness* 68, 69). They transfer the guilt associated with cancer victims onto the viewers themselves—at first shaming the audience by the intimacy they inflict, then aiming to obliterate the distances between the work, the artist, and the audience.

And yet, in spite of their harsh "realism," the photographs are not merely snapshots of reality, Barthes' "message without a code" ("The Photographic Message" 19), but also constructed representations, carefully selected from the hundreds of slides Wilke and Donald Goddard had taken when she entered the hospital in 1991 (Goddard 16). They thus pursue Wilke's lifelong interest in performance art, where the body is the medium by which the subject of art is made visible, both preserving and perverting performance art's form as an unstable site between theater and picture that crucially depends on the presence of an audience. What we know of Wilke's private history obviously inhibits the degree to which we can refer to these photographs as "art"; the illusive dimension of performance art is gruesomely undermined. Yet the work they do in transforming spectators from witnesses into voyeurs and finally into aware participants depends on Wilke's own bodily transformation, and, in this sense, it pursues the aim of performance art to erase the boundary between art and life.

Unlike Spence's double ideological purpose of demystifying the structure of power that produces the diseased body and offering an alternative to the orthodox treatment of cancer, Wilke's photographs do not criticize the kind or quality of the medical treatment she has received. Her critique is directed, rather, toward the act of interpretation itself and its interrelated aesthetic and ethical consequences. Her illness photographs juxtapose traditional pictorial values and cultural conventions with visual marks of disease and treatment, thereby producing a jarring constellation of "constructed" and "real" effects that compels the audience to attend at once to the framed subject/object and to her struggle with cancer, which

THE INVADING BODY

continues beyond and will be determined outside the picture's spatial frame. The sense of urgency and of consequences beyond what is "shown" or "seen" tie the images to an extraphotographic reality in a way that recalls Spence's previously discussed *Marked Up for Amputation* photograph. However, Spence's referral to extraphotographic reality is directly associated with her resistance to the authority of the medical establishment and her attempt to reinstate her autonomy and self-control. By contrast, Wilke's photographs question the possibility of an authentic, resisting self. They replace the duality of subject and object with an exploration of the way in which our very perception of the physical symptoms of disease works in collaboration with prevalent cultural assumptions about illness to undermine the subject's sense of agency. And yet, the audience's guilty awareness of being moved by her art at the expense of her life may be the ultimate performative sign of Wilke's success in re-embodying, embracing, and, thus, affirming her idiosyncratic experience of terminal illness.

In spite of their different emphases, Wilke's and Spence's photographs share an interest in embedding the changed, abject, sick body within the discourse of autobiographical representation. What is at stake in their work is the possibility of broadening the boundaries of the self-documentary mode and, thus, of affecting our perception of what it means to be human. In this sense, their photographs enact Judith Butler's postulation of "the construction of the human as a differential operation" (8). In *Bodies That Matter* Butler underlines the processes of erasure and foreclosure that bind the subject, as it were, from the "outside," forming "an ontological thereness that exceeds or counters" the subject's discursive borders (8). These "excluded sites" haunting the boundaries of discursive legitimacy are at the same time the subject's "constitutive outside" insofar as they have the power to affect and to produce, by disruption and re-articulation, "the more and the less 'human,' the inhuman, the humanly unthinkable" (8). Butler's inquiry into the constitutive force of exclusion usefully applies to the dynamic processes of production and reception through which Wilke's and Spence's self-portraits of illness earn their testimonial significance.[1] In visualizing the experience of terminal illness, their photographs not only resist the reductive force of the biomedical model but also both reiterate and negotiate the boundaries between the culturally legitimate and the culturally refused.

As the chapter on Spence also suggests, the process of granting the sick subject discursive legitimacy beyond the biophysical domain is both rhetorical and collaborative. In eliciting the photograph's testimonial force, Spence and Wilke rely on the performative function of the viewers who help to effect it. If the indexical elements in their photographs—the physical scars that cannot be erased, the transfigured, bloated, or emaciated body—evidently fall short of providing a transparent transcript of the artists' lived experience of illness, they also intensify the photographs' reality effect and, as it were, construct it from the outside through the audience's understanding that not all has been presented, that more acute fears, abjection, and pain have been erased and excluded from the possibility of representation. Lived experience or extraphotographic reality thus meet our imaginative perception insofar as the sick subjects in these photographs are constructed by the excluded possibility of further pain, violent change, and bodily and mental deterioration that exist beyond the photograph's spatial frame and yet can be thought of only in relation to that frame as inhabiting a temporal dimension.

The constant vacillation between spatial arrangements and temporal sequences, which implicates the audience in the reality effect of these photographs, distinguishes Spence's and Wilke's autobiographical work from the growing body of photographs of victorious recovery that explicitly intend to oppose the culturally ingrained beliefs about the ill as dehumanized, deformed and—especially in the case of breast cancer—desexualized victims of disease. The following discussion of self-portraits by Ariela Shavid and photographs of women who have survived breast cancer by Art Myers shows that the desire to embed cancer survivors within available discourses of cultural legitimacy may ironically result in the photographic denial of the reality of sickness. In contrast with Spence and Wilke, both Shavid and Myers attain social reintegration and inclusion by minimizing and, when possible, excluding from the pictures those indexical elements that would enable the viewers to invest the images in a temporal sequence of illness. Arguably, their images can be "read," as all images can be, but the stories they tell have been separated from the photographed subjects' experience of illness in a way that comes to occlude, too, their experience of recovery. Shavid's photographs are engaged in a critique of gender roles and, more particularly, of the entrenched causal connection between women's beauty and their happiness. Her images provide meta-stories about the cultural production of approved body images in a patriarchal consumer society. Myers's photographs, for their part, celebrate the persistence of female beauty by visualizing normative scenes and episodes that only accidentally feature cancer survivors. It is the effort to negate the experiential difference between the sick and the healthy that ultimately contradicts the explicit ideological goal in these photographs of representing cancer survivors as legitimate members of society.

Thus, Shavid's untitled self-portraits in figure 15, from a series of fourteen works originally assembled and exhibited as a copybook, in no way lend themselves to a reading of the individual's experience of illness. In fact, even to treat them as self-portraits is problematic since the identities that they suggest—the film star or glamorous hostess, the student, the bride—are so obviously a function of the poses and various costumes Shavid assumes, the artificiality of which is further enhanced by the broken lines that identify the photographed figures as paper dolls.

Granted, as Roee Rosen has pointed out, "the exposure of a personal truth in these photographs—in the most factual sense, since the presence of the no-breast is a symptom of a malignant disease, irreversible, coerced, dangerous and threatening—will not allow us to comfortably classify it beside [Cindy] Sherman's early works" (2). This valid alert to the special status of even the most "postmodern" of illness photographs should not, however, be taken to apply to all illness photographs in the same way. While the personal disclosure of Shavid's injured body may heighten the series' cultural critique, her amputated breast, too, is duplicated in the pictures by the same objectifying strategies of repetition and framing that suggest the stereotypic production of women as desirable objects in patriarchal mass culture. In other words, rather than draw attention to the experience of one's body as irreplaceable and unique, the lack of perfection that the missing breast signifies serves here to parody the reiterative

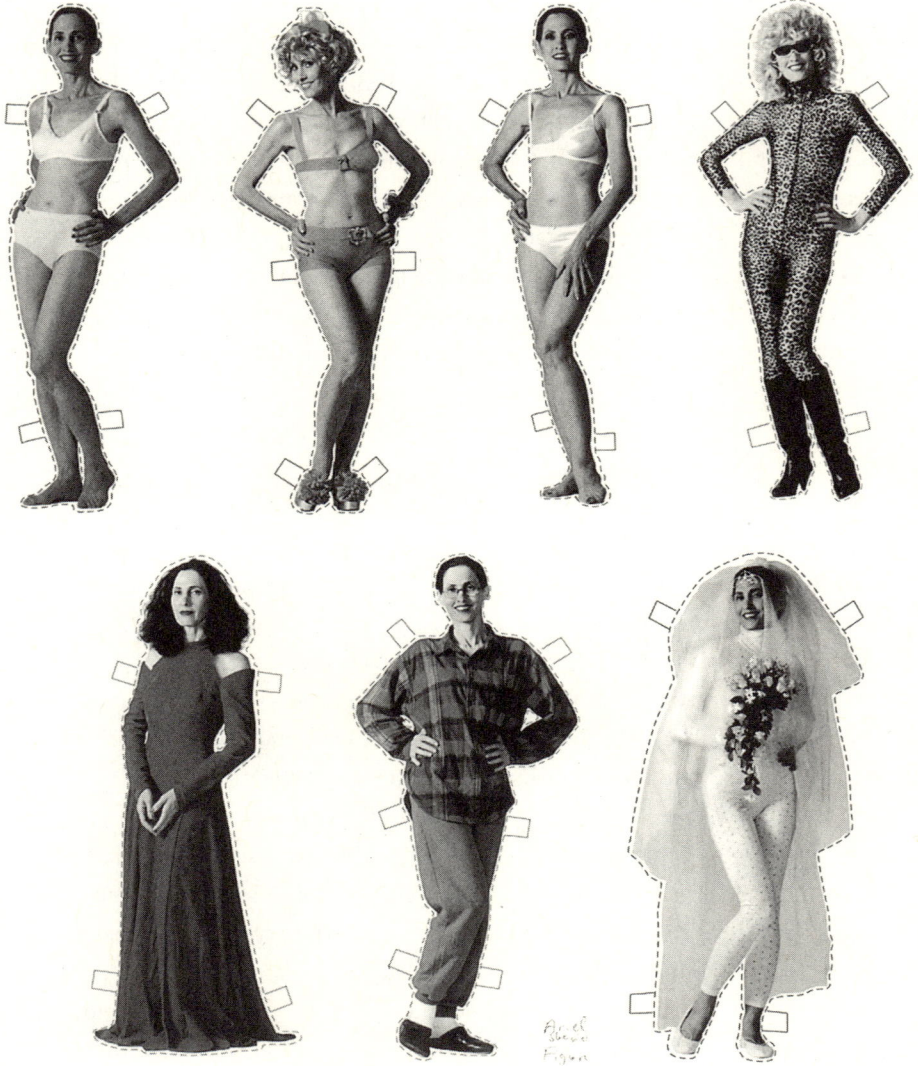

Figure 15. Ariela Shavid, *"Beauty Is a Promise of Happiness."* 1996. (Seven color photographs, computer prints, 95 x 70 cm, from a series of 14 works assembled and exhibited as a copybook. Copyright 1996 Ariela Shavid. Courtesy of the artist.)

mechanisms of desire and their economic mobilization in late capitalism. In this sense Shavid has indeed incorporated her wounded body in a social criticism that equally applies to the healthy and the sick. Yet, her success in making deformity legitimate relies on an implicit equation between one's experience of surviving cancer and any other culturally constituted lack. Such a structuralist equation inevitably dilutes and suppresses the temporal and embodied dimensions of the personal experiences of illness and recovery. Ironically, by including the one-breasted woman within the feminist critique of the masculine gaze—by counting her within the normative category of "women"—Shavid must pay the symbolic price of repudiating the experiential dimensions of illness and pain, a repudiation that, in Butler's terms, demands their simultaneous production as abject, "'unlivable' and 'uninhabitable' zones of social life" (3).

Shavid's satirical recruitment of advertising strategies such as fashion styling, careful staging, enlargement, and duplication as a way of exposing the cultural practices that construct sex as a fantasy is very different indeed from Art Myers's candid celebration of female beauty in his photographs of breast-cancer survivors. A physician and self-educated art photographer, Myers's professional and personal encounters with breast cancer have required him to confront the prevalent unease about sexuality shared by cancer survivors and their partners.[2] These encounters motivated him "to show that a woman's fundamental nature is not dependent on anything external; the loss of part or all of her breast is not a threat to her being" (Preface). His photographic project includes short narratives written by the photographed women and their partners, as well as poems and "fine art" photography, an example of which can be seen in figure 16, which appears on the book's cover. His hope, he says, is that "these pictures, poems and personal vignettes will reveal the persistence of a woman's beauty, strength and femaleness in all of its complexity, even after the transforming experience of breast cancer" (Preface).

It is the persistence of a woman's beauty that is presumably represented in figure 16 by the organic images of bird and tree that visually embed the female body in a matrix of traditional connotations. This might be an image of Daphne in the midst of transforming herself into a tree—unproblematically aligned with the visual patterns of the genre of the female

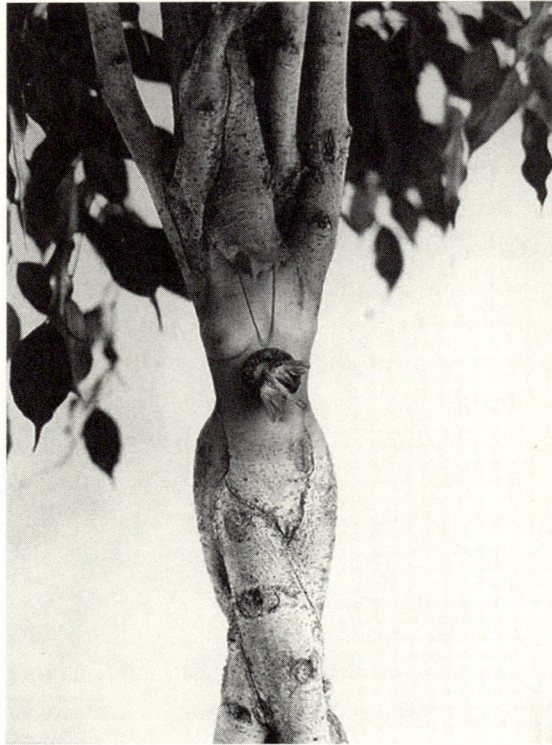

Figure 16. Art Myers, *Sometimes a Leaf Will Fall before Autumn*. (Copyright 1996 by Art Myers. Courtesy of the artist.)

nude, such as the conventional association of Woman with Nature and of Woman's nudity with an alluring sexuality characterized by unthreatening passivity. The picture has been manipulated to render the place where the amputated breast once was as smooth and unobtrusive as the merging joints where the woman's body ingeniously fades into tree trunk and branches. One can understand how the photograph may serve Myers's purpose of opposing the culturally ingrained assumption "that a perfect breast is the requisite icon of the feminine essence" (Preface). Arguably, however, the "feminine essence" he wants to show that even a one-breasted woman can have seems very close to what Gill Saunders has defined as "the exhibitionism and narcissism, the vulnerability and victimization" (24) of the classical nude model.[3]

THE INVADING BODY

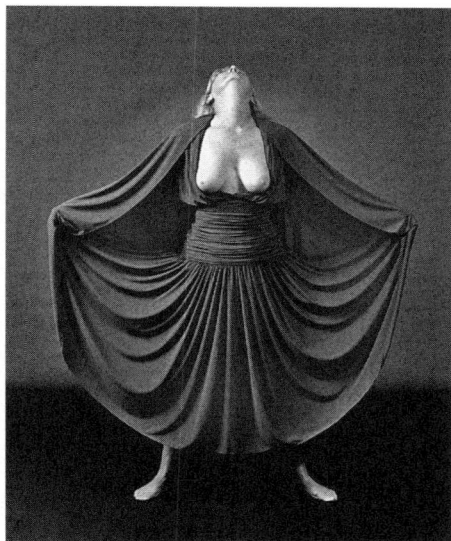

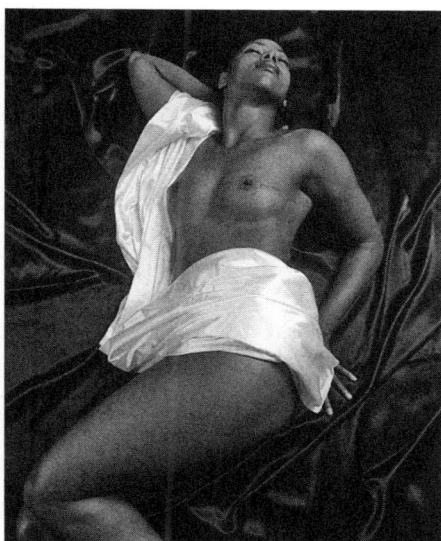

Figures 17 and 18. Art Myers, *Stephanie* and *Yavonne*. (Copyright 1996 by Art Myers. Courtesy of the artist.)

Unwittingly, perhaps, not only Myers's anonymous "artistic" nudes but also his photographs of breast cancer survivors conform to the rules of the genre. The photographs of Yavonne (figure 18) and of his wife, Stephanie (figure 17), are a case in point: in both of these photographs the woman's eyes are averted while her body, to borrow Saunders's phrase, "is displayed to the gaze of the viewer, the pose carefully contrived so as not to interfere with his visual access" (24). In these photographs, the indexical signs of disease have been eliminated to such a degree that the images might indeed appease the anxiety of both cancer victims and viewers about the sexuality of the sick. The ability to interpolate these women as traditional nude models and the erotic pleasure ensured by the spectacle are themselves the most effective signs of the normative sexuality of the women portrayed.

Yet, if the domain of the abject has been humanized by exclusion, that is, through the repudiation of any sign of disease from the normative display of conventionally construed sexuality, the autobiographical texts that accompany the images resist the pictorial message. The short narrative beside Yavonne's picture reads: "An important part of going through my breast cancer experience was the fact that it did not make me feel unattractive or take away the sensual feelings about myself.—Yavonne." This self-assured, self-asserting testimony of having had "sensual feelings about myself" while experiencing cancer is clearly incongruous with Yavonne's pictorial rendition in terms of the voyeuristic generic conventions of the female nude.

The autobiographical affirmation of the legitimacy of the relation of sexuality and illness has been erased from the image, which strives, rather, to obliterate or at least blur the indexical mark of illness through soft "erotic" lighting and a carefully contrived pose that hides the asymmetry between the reconstructed and the healthy breast. Significantly, the photographic strategies used to produce "Yavonne" are the same as those used in the traditional erotic depiction of female nakedness for male consumption. As a result, the autobiographical demand for a self-empowering sensuality that survives the experience of cancer, where one not only feels attractive but has sensual feelings about *herself,* has been replaced in the photograph with the conventional passive and objectifying sleeping pose.[4]

The disruption posed by the incongruity between the photograph and the accompanying autobiographical text is even more acutely felt in Stephanie's portrait. The photograph shows her dancing in a low-cut dress that centers the viewer's attention on her exposed breasts. Her feet are bare and her head is thrown back ecstatically, suggesting her immersion in this moment of physical pleasure. Nearly all the conventions of the nude genre have been met here: the contrived display, the averted glance, the wantonness and narcissism. However, the narrative next to the photograph reads:

The mammograms were negative and the doctors assured me there was nothing to worry about. However, the quarter-sized lump in my right breast turned out to be cancer. My breast and right arm took quite a beating after the lympectomy, lymphadenectomy, surgery, radiation, and radioactive implants. Over time my breast has again become fairly symmetrical. Now the solid mass on the outer side of my breast and the occasional ache and swelling in my arm remind me how precious each day is.—Stephanie

THE INVADING BODY

The overwhelming personal history of tests, false results, further testing, diagnosis, prolonged and painful treatment, and the diverse emotional reaction to each phase in the ongoing crisis is totally absent from the photograph. Even the reference to her precarious physical and emotional well-being in the present has been excluded. Her occasionally swollen and aching arm is carefully covered by her dress; the gnawing bodily awareness of the preciousness of each day translated into a pose of erotic abandon. Ironically, the only agreement between word and image here is implied by the phrase "[o]ver time my breast has again become fairly symmetrical," a phrase that, although it finds its pictorial correspondence in the photograph, nonetheless undermines Myers's previously quoted claim to critique the cultural maxim that "a perfect breast is the requisite icon of the feminine essence."

Rather than highlight the legitimacy of the relation between illness and sexuality in any significant way, these photographs not only reiterate the traditional patriarchal devices that produce women as sexual objects but in fact rely on their pictorial expression as a way of repudiating the subjects' history of illness. Granted, not all the photographs in the book follow the same pattern, but all more or less consistently aspire to present the women's "transcendence" of breast cancer by situating them in settings that deny the difficulties of illness, remission, and recovery. Many photographs tell small "humane" stories of love, professional success, and recreational hobbies that are meant to counterbalance the literal message of the women's mastectomy scars. By staging, thus, the subjects' lives in the present, the pictures endeavor to show cancer survivors not as victims—indeed not as sick people at all. And yet, in negating the experience of illness as a formative personal narrative, and in excluding from the photographs the crucial experiential differences between illness and remission, and remission and recovery, the photographs also totally erase the survivors' conceivable worries about illness in the present, most poignantly the constant awareness of the possibility of a recurrence.

By contrast, the autobiographical projects of Spence and Wilke engage in cultural work that empowers them as embodied subjects at the same time that they negotiate our reception of the cultural and medical meanings of serious illness. These two concerns—working "inward" and "outward"—distinguish their work from the tradition of documentary photography, as well as from the great corpus of postmodernist photographs that seek to collapse the distinction between reality and phantasm. Autobiographical illness photographs differ from traditional documentation since they are usually constructed by the subjects of photography themselves, who direct or even stage (previsualize) the shooting and, when technically possible, press the shutter ("take" the pictures) themselves. By intentionally blurring the boundaries between subject and object, they evade the often demeaning and distorting subject-object relation characteristic of the photographic documentary mode.[5] A conscious confusion of subject and object is, of course, one of the hallmarks of postmodernist photography. Yet, while illness photographs may employ postmodernist aesthetics in ways that expose the constructed process of their composition, their indexical references to embodied suffering are clearly not fantasized for the sake of an artistic declaration. Postmodern photographers, such as Cindy Sherman, have been celebrated not merely for working with, parodying, and citing the culturally givens—they are hailed for collapsing the distinction between the subject and object of photography, thereby canceling the possibility of distinguishing between the actual and the simulated. Their work, as Rosalind Krauss has put it, "functions as a refusal to understand the artist as a source of originality, a fount of subjective response" (22). By contrast, autobiographical illness photographs foreground the artist's visualization of her illness both in terms of the body's intentionality—its lived dimension—and as it is seen through cultural and biomedical lenses, as malleable, fashionable, diagnosable, and treatable. They are inevitably subjective yet intensely real responses to the experience of suffering, often made in conscious opposition to the passive role imposed on the photographer by her culture's narratives and the medical establishment.

Autobiographical illness photographs are, therefore, inconsistent with the critical category of postmodernist photography, inasmuch as they are not constrained by the definitive or prototypical feature of postmodernist photographs: the attempt to frustrate and refute the viewer's assumption of a prephotographic reality to which the photographs refer.[6] As we have seen, even in illness photographs whose postmodernist orientation makes the symbolic message explicit by formal means of irony and even of par-

THE INVADING BODY

ody, their indexical, denoted message offers an oppositional force that pulls the viewer's attention away from the deliberately symbolic, contrived, and manipulated meaning and balances it against a sense of truth-value and of real consequences beyond the photograph's frame. Thus, Wilke may pose as a playboy bunny, Holy Mother, or a character in a horror film, but the bandages on her neck forcefully undermine her playful engagement with cultural citations. The powerful reality effect of Spence's staged tableaux is, similarly, inextricable from our operational knowledge of her illness, which is triggered, and yet not exhausted, by her juxtaposition of hospital-ward photographs with those that show her receiving alternative treatment.

The particular form of perception illness photographs compel re-invokes the sense of a real referent that dominates photography, which has been almost unanimously discarded from the theoretical inquiries into the medium of photography in the last three decades. Since Allan Secula published his groundbreaking essay "On the Invention of Photographic Meaning" in 1975, and even more so since the publication of Barthes' "Rhetoric of the Image" in 1978, reading photographs as complex cultural messages has gradually become the normative critical approach. Critics such as Douglas Crimp, Rosalind Krauss, Martha Rosler, Abigail Solomon-Godeau, and John Tagg, well-read in semiotic, post-structuralist, and feminist literature, have posed such questions as why certain photographic images are made, and to what ends they are put by those who commission them. Following Barthes' and Secula's initial undertaking, these critics have productively analyzed the cultural and political signification of photographic connotations, and theorized about the ideological meaning that inheres in the mechanical apparatus of the camera itself. From this perspective, the photograph's inevitably exclusive and reductive frame of reference reflects a process of selection and editing that, as Graham Clarke has pointed out, ensures "the recapitulation not so much of an objective reality, as of a subject framed by a set of ideological assumptions and values" (23). Postmodernist photography, in its overt articulation of the constructed and the simulated, has been stamped as the standard representative prototype against which the medium of photography as a category is to be measured and described.

Yet, as has been my argument throughout, the extremity of autobiographical illness photographs—their "non-focalness" within photography as a category—calls for a test of the descriptions of the category.[7] In the tradition of photographic theory, these descriptions center almost exclusively on the relation of photography and language. The two conventional descriptions of this relationship have been identified by W. J. T. Mitchell as "fundamentally antithetical": the first stresses photography's difference from language, characterizing it as "'a message without a code', a purely objective transcript of visual reality"; while the second "turns photography into a language, or stresses its absorption by language in actual use" (282). Following Barthes, Mitchell accounts for these conflicting descriptions in terms of the "photographic paradox," "the co-existence of two messages, the one without a code (the photographic analogue), the other with a code (the 'art', or the treatment or the 'writing', or the rhetoric of the photograph" (Barthes, "The Photographic Message" 19; qtd. in Mitchell 284).

Mitchell realizes, however, that the photographic paradox is not resolved but rather restated by the structural division of photography into connotative and denotative levels of signification:

One connotation always present in the photograph is that it is a pure denotation; that is simply what it means to recognize it as a photograph rather than some other sort of image. Conversely, the denotation of a photograph, what we take it to represent, is never free from what we take it to mean. . . . Connotation goes all the way down to the roots of the photograph, to the motives for its production, to the selection of its subject matter, to the choice of angles and lighting. Similarly, "pure denotation" reaches all the way up to the most textually "readable" features of the photograph: the photograph is "read" as if it were the trace of an event. (284)

Intrinsic to photography is an element of pure spectatorship that defies rhetoric, if rhetoric is defined as meaning produced by an investment of values. This is why Barthes posits photography as a site of "resistance" to

THE INVADING BODY

rhetoric (Mitchell 285). Yet elsewhere Barthes makes clear that we never encounter this visually literal element of photography "in its pure state"—rather, we can only trace its effects as it "naturalizes the symbolic message, [and] innocents the semantic artifice of connotation" ("Rhetoric of the Image" 276, 279).

The current categorical description of photography as textuality, albeit in a different modality than that of verbal texts, has rendered Barthes' concept of the photographic paradox irrelevant and obsolete. As the critical pendulum swings decisively in favor of treating photography just like any other (cultural) text, even critics who continue to use Barthes' terms *denotation* and *connotation* insist that the facade of the photographic paradox has been happily exposed by our greater understanding of the mechanisms that help to effect it.[8] A rare contestant to this constructionist description is Christian Metz in "Photography and Fetish." Metz draws on Charles Sanders Peirce's terms *index, icon,* and *symbol* in order to emphasize the special status of photography as a mode of expression that is fundamentally indexical. "Peirce," he says, "called indexical the process of signification . . . in which the signifier is bound to the referent not by a social convention (= 'symbol'), not necessarily by some similarity (= 'icon'), but by an actual contiguity or connection in the world" (156). According to Metz, what is indexical about photography is "the mode of production itself, the principle of the taking" (156). However, the indexical elements of photography (the physical and chemical marks of its making) have been problematized if not altogether annulled by the prevailing critical discourse, which privileges the more "readable" iconic and symbolic aspects.

By suggesting that indexical elements invade the photograph's most textual level, Metz in fact reiterates Barthes' idea of the photographic paradox. While I doubt that such indexicality can be accounted for in every photograph, Spence's and Wilke's examples of autobiographical illness photographs clearly contain a gradient of indexical elements that calls for a re-evaluation of Barthes' concept of the photographic paradox and a rereading of his formulation of the relation of photography and time. Barthes' discarded concepts are more useful explanatory tools than those supplied by the strong constructivist approach, which fails to acknowledge the nondetermined boundaries of the category of photography and evaluate the category directly by its prototypes as (only) a construction.

In his "Rhetoric of the Image" Barthes has argued that at the literal level of the photograph, "the relationship of signifieds to signifiers is not one of 'transformation' but of 'recording'" (278). In *Camera Lucida,* published two years later, he already feels obliged to fend off criticism of his allegedly dated realist position. The following passage from *Camera Lucida* (published in 1980) continues to attract critical altercation today.

It is the fashion, nowadays, among Photography's commentators . . . to seize upon a semantic relativity: no "reality" (great scorn for the "realists" who do not see that the photograph is always coded), nothing but artifice: *Thesis,* not *Physis;* the Photograph, they say, is not an *analogon* of the world; what it represents is fabricated, because the photographic optic is subject to Albertian perspective (entirely historical) and because the inscription on the picture makes a three-dimensional object into a two-dimensional effigy. This argument is futile: nothing can prevent the Photograph from being analogical; but at the same time, Photography's noeme has nothing to do with analogy (a feature it shares with all kinds of representation). The realists, of whom I am one and of whom I was already one when I asserted that the Photograph was an image without code—even if, obviously, certain codes do inflect our reading of it—the realists do not take the photograph for a "copy" of reality, but for an emanation of *past reality: a magic,* not an art. (88)

What has changed from "Rhetoric" to *Camera Lucida* is not so much Barthes' punctuated insistence on the photograph's analogical functions as his rephrasing of the literal message of the image in terms of its power to bear testimony "not on the object but on time" (89). If, in "Rhetoric," much attention was devoted to the cultural and symbolically readable elements of the image, in *Camera,* Barthes highlights the contingent, indexical, deictic elements—the "absolute Particular" or "This" each photograph "mechanically repeats" but that "could never be repeated existentially" (4). Perhaps, as has been suggested by critics, Barthes' celebration of the photograph's particularity as magic has to be read against the death of his mother and "his search for 'a just image' and not 'just an image' of her" (Tagg 1).⁹ *Camera* is certainly a personal monument, a moving gesture of mourning that quite explicitly sets out to tell more of Barthes as son and writer than of photography at large. It seems to me, however, equally plausible that Barthes concentrated on the contingent elements of photography because, as he acknowledges in the previously quoted passage, the changed critical climate around him had rendered superfluous the repetition of those cultural and semiotic meaning-making aspects on which he enlarged in his "Rhetoric."

In "Rhetoric," the notion of the photographic paradox suggested a structural balance between the image's denotative and connotative meanings, so that its referential force was checked (and in its pure form rendered utopian) by its culturally coded construction. In *Camera* Barthes attempts to circumvent this conceptual standstill by arguing that, regardless of any "fabrication" (staging) of the image or a deflection of its meaning owing to the medium's built-in mechanisms, the photograph authenticates the viewer's sense of the passing of time. Thus, he states, "[t]he important thing is that the photograph possesses an evidential force, and that its testimony bears not on the object but on time. From a phenomenological viewpoint, in the Photograph, the power of authentication exceeds the power of representation" (*Camera* 89).

In the light of the poststructuralist and new historicist insights of the last three decades it is not easy to naively embrace this passage's strong phenomenological vocabulary, even though much available evidence from the text of *Camera* itself contradicts its essentialist thrust. Critics such as John Tagg have made these two sentences the butt of their intellectual scorn, accusing Barthes not only of employing simplistic notion of "retrospective realism" but also, more subtly, of giving voice to the "nostalgic and regressive phantasy" (4) of a whole critical generation that mouthed but could not quite digest the implications of the signifier's severance from the signified. At every stage of the photograph's production, says Tagg,

> chance effects, purposeful interventions, choices and variations produce meaning, whatever skill is applied and whatever division of labour the process is subject to. This is not the inflection of a prior (though irretrievable) reality, as Barthes would have us believe, but the production of a new and specific reality, the photograph, which becomes meaningful in certain transactions and has real effects, but which cannot refer or be referred to a pre-photographic reality as to a truth. (3)

Furthermore, "the very idea of what constitutes evidence has a history— a history which has escaped Barthes" (4). Accordingly, "what Barthes calls 'evidential force' is a complex historical outcome and is exercised by photographs only within certain institutional practices and within particular historical relations" (4).

Yet, a reading of *Camera* as a whole makes clear that when Barthes speaks of photographic "authentication," he is not claiming that it is an inherent photographic trait but rather an effect particular details in specific photographs have vis-à-vis a specific viewer. Notwithstanding Tagg's persuasive description of photographic production, his reading strangely suppresses Barthes' articulation of the audience's position and is therefore unjust to Barthes' complex thought. Embarrassingly, Tagg's own definition of the photograph's "real" meaning as that which includes "not just the material item but also the discursive system of which the image it bears is part" (4) is a repetition of Barthes' idea of photographic connotations as expressed in "Rhetoric of the Image," published ten years earlier. By reductively identifying the whole of Barthes' thought on the issue with a single passage from *Camera,* Tagg erases Barthes' enormous contribution to our very ability to speak so fluently of "the discursive system of the image" and, even more, to our ability to think of photography's "reality effect" as "an effect of the production of the subject in and through representation" (Tagg 4).

In analyzing the reality effect of autobiographical illness photographs,

I have, thus, built on Barthes' idea of the collaborative role of the audience as a primarily interactive and interconstitutive process of authentication. More specifically, this discussion has shown that our operational knowledge of the presence of what Barthes defined as "literal message" (our sense that "this is how it was") has performative consequences that compel a particular form of perception. The literal message does not contribute to the photograph's reality effect merely by, as has been quoted before, "[naturalizing] the symbolic message" ("Rhetoric" 279). This holds true for "realistic" photographs, photographs that are invested in affecting verisimilitude, but the denotative message has a somewhat different function in the "postmodern" illness photographs that this and the previous chapters have explored. In Spence's and Wilke's staged and previsualized photographs, the denoted message actively subverts the spatially constructed iconic and symbolic meanings by displacing/shifting the evidential force of the photographs from the subject of the image to the audience's sense of time. The temporal dimension that has been, thus, introduced, deictically refers the audience to the artists' pre- and postphotographic reality of terminal illness.

Extraphotographic reality emerges, too, when we attend to the dynamic processes of production and reception that implicate the images we see in the idiosyncrasies of the photographer's lived experience of illness and of her simultaneous engagement in the representation of illness. In the discussion of Spence's cancer photographs in particular, I have replaced Barthes' phenomenological emphasis with an emphasis on the processes of photographic production and reception. These dynamic processes better explain the reality effect of illness photographs since they both account for the rhetorically constructed position of the audience in illness photographs and steer away from the monolithic, universal subject of traditional phenomenology that has been effectively deconstructed in the last decades by various poststructuralist approaches. Still, Barthes' idea that the photograph testifies to the passing of time has rich implications not only in regard to an examination of illness photographs but also for my perception (elaborated in the previous chapters) of the truth-value of illness narratives as a temporal process that emerges in the act of writing and its reception. Autobiographical illness photographs share with personal illness narratives a persistent evidential force that testifies to the inadequacy of the received descriptions of photographic and verbal autobiographies as wholly constructed and absorbed by constitutive, nonreferential patterns. By demanding the collaboration of their audience to effect the emergence of the individual's voice at the site of physical crisis, illness photographs and illness narratives resist the strong constructivist canons that conceive of the categories of photography and narrative only in terms of prior discursive practices.

THE INVADING BODY

CONCLUSION

THE INVESTIGATION OF AUTOBIOGRAPHICAL ILLNESS NARRA-
tives and photographs in this book has emphasized the relation between
the conventional patterns through which the body is objectified in self-
representational practices and the deictic elements in the texts and works
that not only point at but are themselves contingent on concrete conditions of embodied experience. While each chapter has explored different
aspects of the production, address, and reception of personal accounts of
illness, when taken together, they confirm the special status of this new
genre in light of its unique enactment of a gradient of relations between
the discursive and the experientially contingent. I have argued that the
existence of a combination of contiguous and constructed elements in
illness narratives transgresses the current constructionist descriptions of
autobiography and places the subgenre, as a nonfocal case, at the boundaries of the category of autobiographical writing. Similarly, autobiographical illness photographs have been shown as capable of testing and problematizing the dominant cultural constructionist view of photography
as textuality.

A governing hypothesis in the book has been my conviction that, since
illness narratives and photographs are intensely engaged in enacting and
thematizing the body as a constellation of objectified and experiential
states of being, they have valuable contributions to make to the contem-

porary scholarly preoccupation with processes of embodiment and materialization. My discussion of specific texts and works has demonstrated that the multileveled crisis of a major illness and the experience of living with bodily limitations generate both the sensation and the realization that lived experience is not only about living in objectified bodies, as cultural constructionists would lead us to think.[1] All the writers and photographers whose work I examined present their embodied experience of illness as a process of learning to recognize bodily sensations as valid and forceful knowledge. Their narratives and photographs provide concrete examples of the intersection and dialectic interaction of embodied knowledge with literary and cultural forms of knowledge in the historically situated project of personal meaning-making.

This is not to say, however, that all illness narratives and photographs envision the experience of illness as a process of learning, or, indeed, that there is or should be a finite goal to that process. The variegated testimonies in this book alone defy such an abstract teleological framework. Surely, moreover, my own inclinations as well as my selection of texts and works also influenced the paradigm of learning that organizes the direction of this discussion. Out of the vast, and quickly growing, body of illness narratives and photographs that has flourished since the 1960s, my own selection was rather homogenous in the sense that it encompassed narratives and photographs written and produced by writers and artists already established in other, more literary genres, such as poetry and fiction, or else engaged in academic writing, journalism, editing, and professional photography. All of the texts and photographs were written and produced specifically for publication, that is, with an audience and purpose in mind other than writing and taking photographs only for oneself or for one's close circle of family members and friends. In fact, excepting Audre Lorde and, to some extent, Jo Spence, the texts and works discussed in this book fit G. Thomas Couser's observation in respect to the racial and class hegemony of illness and disability narratives (*Recovering* 4).

It remains to future research to explore the social, political, and economic conditions of race and class and the ways in which they are inscribed in the experiencing, ailing body. One crucial consequence of the

THE INVADING BODY

racial and class homogeneity of the autobiographical illness narratives and photographs I have discussed seems rather obvious. I refer, of course, to the writers' and photographers' substantial economical privileges. Predominantly white and middle-class professionals, the writers and photographers whose work I have examined had access to the best available orthodox and alternative health care, and were free of the need to continue to work while undergoing treatment for fear of losing their health insurance. In this sense, they were concretely armored against the horrendous social and medical conditions of the less-privileged sick by their income, investments, health insurance, and private ability to pay for life-extending procedures, such as bone marrow transplants, which are usually refused coverage by insurance companies. Social and economic differences have, therefore, a direct bearing on the primary characteristic of the body as material activity, which includes the basic material conditions of treatment as well as the material access to privileged practices of self-representation. Although autobiography has been identified as the most democratic of literary genres (Howells 798), future investigation of testimonies of illness produced by people of more diverse racial and social affiliations may begin by examining the material political-economic conditions of marginalized individuals and groups and the ways these affect and effect the experience of illness as well as the accessibility of the autobiographical genre.

Other directions for future study are suggested by illness autobiographies' perception of the experiencing body as both subject and object. I believe that our cultural understanding of the malleability and irreducibility of the corporeal self would be enriched rather than obscured by new biomedical research into the functioning of the brain, itself described by neurologists as a peculiar amalgam of theory and flesh. While feminist scholars at the front line of embodiment theory tend to privilege psychoanalytical paradigms over biomedical and other "scientific" models, which they view as ideologically biased by essentialist assumptions, I believe we have much to learn from contemporary cognitive and neurological studies of memory and learning processes. Poststructuralist, feminist, and culturalist critics have more interests in common with current developments in biomedical studies than they care to acknowledge, since even science and technology studies today criticize the long-held notion that the body, and nature, as an object of research can be "discovered" by scientific research.[2] Ironically, while this classical notion remains a favorite target of attack in the humanities,[3] recent studies in evolutionary and neurobiology and in the field known as bioepistemology actually promote models of brain work that embed postmodernist values such as fluidity and malleability, even though they tie them to natural constraints; for example, an innate human preference for patterns that facilitates our ability to remember and learn.[4] I find it truly amazing that prominent scholars in poststructuralist embodiment theory, such as Grosz and Weiss, refrain from consulting these new resources and continue to rely on dated neurophysiological research, a great part of which Schilder and Merleau-Ponty used to support their own conceptualizations of the embodied subject in the first half of the twentieth century.

A fascinating and promising arena for an interdisciplinary inquiry that would combine the study of self-reflexive and self-representative practices with recent cognitive and neurophysiological paradigms might pursue, as a model, John Sutton's work on memory and epistemology. Sutton's assumption, based on recent neurological and cognitive research, is that memory traces in the brain are not "local, independent atoms which faithfully store and reproduce the past" (281). The model he adheres to is not that of an archive or a library. Rather, he describes memory in terms of distributed neural patterns, where new memory inputs are superimposed on the same processing network and are inevitably affected by traces of previously stored patterns. The resulting mixture between the traces of earlier patterns and the new input is what the network remembers. In a nutshell, Sutton claims that memory by definition is always reconstructive. We do not have direct access to the past since memories are not encoded as complete units to be later retrieved as in storehouse models—memory traces are not event-analogues or literal copies of the structure of experience. They are both interest-determined and interest-carried, structured by multiple contexts of retention and recall. Furthermore, "we tell more than we remember: later inferences creep into the telling" (Sutton 308). Accordingly, as we verbalize our memories, the trace

THE INVADING BODY

of an event is likely to be filtered through other—later—beliefs, dreams, fears, or wishes.

Yet, the reconstructive nature of remembering does not mean that the past is "obstructed" or "distorted" by a veil of representations (i.e., patterns by which memory traces are organized in the brain). To assume that would necessarily also assume a threefold structure of perception including reality "out there," representations, and the subject who is either blinded by or seeing through representations. Sutton claims that, in fact, there is no transparent reality, or indeed a central internal interpreter—the subject. All we have, in all of our encounters with reality, are representations and new inputs, in learning as in remembering:

> In distributed models, there is no internal central processor which searches, inspects, or otherwise manipulates items stored passively in discrete memory locations. The only connections within the system are local, and processing and storage occur in the same parts of the system. . . . Behaviour mediated by cognitive activity is the result not of an intelligent homunculus' calculations, but of numerous relatively independent but interacting systems computing best-fit solutions in parallel. (Sutton 313)

New work drawing from the distributed neural model in reading illness autobiographies and, indeed, in studying other self-representational practices, would underscore the biological basis of human behavior and knowledge. Once we accept the unity of brain and mind, we can begin to explore the dynamic relations among lived experience, the ways the brain organizes and processes inputs and patterns, and the ways in which memories and the remembering subject are produced in discourse. The inherently reconstructive nature of memory is a good place to start since it can test the conceptual gap between "real" and narrated experience that has haunted autobiographical studies for the last three decades. We have seen, in chapter 3 of this work, that the deconstructivist and cultural constructionist approaches to memorized personal "truth" reject it as arbitrary and falsified by language or by other cultural institutions. Yet, if what we remember is always a reconstructive mixture of new inputs and previous representations—if this is how our brains work, then the residual polarity in these approaches between true and false, authentic and constructed memories is no longer tenable. Moreover, the presumed perversion of truth entailed by the articulation of lived experience in language also loses its edge when the processes of construction involved in self-writing and the (re)constructed selves that such writing produces are modeled on biological, innate, constraints in addition to cultural and discursive structures.

Illness autobiographies may usefully highlight the constellation of new inputs and representations that structure our "normal" encounters with reality. The crisis of serious illness generates extreme, new experiences and sensations that can break down the habits of a lifetime. Illness narratives dramatize the dynamic interplay between such contiguous sensory inputs and the context-bound processes of internal reconstruction and reorganization, which are affected by the writers' already processed patterns of thought and feeling. Since writers of illness narratives usually divide their experience into pre- and present reality of illness, or conceive of themselves in terms of the current, sick self and the lost, healthy self, it would be interesting to ask which previously established memory patterns are nonetheless mixed with, and thus color, the embodied experience of illness. How, in other words, do earlier patterns serve to either obstruct or preserve the continuity and bodily integrity of the self and, conversely, what role do they play in the self-exertion toward plasticity and learning evidenced in the desire to refashion our bodily condition, to write our own terms for our knowledge of self in the face of the irreducibility of bodily illness?

Nancy Easterlin persuasively argues that "without the inborn tendency to organize information in specific ways, we would not be able to experience choice in our responses. Chaos would take the place of experience, and our species would not have survived" (4). Whether they are inborn or developed early in a social context, or, probably, both, it is important to recognize that our modes of processing and organizing lived experience are not only cultural but also material. The new available resources on brain mechanisms should productively substantiate Elizabeth

Grosz's call in *Volatile Bodies* to explore the material in culture and the cultural in the corporeal. Moreover, they may help us to refine our ability to distinguish between the two modalities of attention demanded by illness narratives, which Arthur Frank has defined as listening to what illness stories say *about* the body and attending to stories as being told *through* the body (2).

An integrative view of Frank's modalities captures what I have been trying to convey through my explorations of illness autobiographies and photographs. The extent to which illness narratives and photographs are contingent on extratextual and extraphotographic circumstances stands in direct relation to their reality effect—the effect of being told and performed through the sick body. Yet extratextual reality itself is not transparent but an intermixture of sensations and structuring patterns. I have looked to traces of the invasion of the body as both embedded within and at the same time excluded from the cultural and discursive constructs by which the body is regulated and objectified. If illness autobiographies and photographs share the generic autobiographical attribute of (re)constructing the embodied self as a discursive object, they also compel us to recognize and affirm the body as an active and constitutive agent of subjectivity.

NOTES

INTRODUCTION

1. Nancy Mairs, *Waist-high in the World;* Robert F. Murphy, *The Body Silent;* Lennard J. Davis, *Bending over Backwards;* Tobin Siebers, "Disability in Theory."

2. In talking of the inadequacy of theoretical discourse on the body, I too employ that very discourse. I am fully aware of the irony of using the current abstract professional discourse on the body at the same time that I attempt to dismantle it, and yet this is what I must do if I wish to respond to and engage in a dialogue with the available contemporary scholarship.

3. The idea of "imaginative identification" engendered by illness narratives parallels and is indeed indebted to Richard Rorty's formulation of the liberal ironist's "ability to envisage and desire to prevent the actual and possible humiliation of others" (93).

4. This concept pursues Arthur W. Frank's idea of experience as a rhetorical process (22). Philippe Lejeune was first to elaborate on this sense of authenticity, not as "the being-in-itself of the past (if indeed such a thing exists), but being-for-itself, manifested in the present of the enunciation" (25).

5. Anne Hunsaker Hawkins was first to use *pathography* to refer to an autobiographical or biographical narrative about an experience of illness. Her description of the history of the usage of the term, first by Freud and later by Oliver Sacks, appears in the notes to the introduction of *Reconstructing Illness* (177–78).

6. Still, Hawkins herself, somewhat inconsistently, devotes all of *Reconstructing Illness* to a detailed taxonomy of the organizing myths and cultural metaphors common in illness narratives.

7. Thus, in his cleverly titled book *Facing It: AIDS Diaries and the Death of the Author,* Ross Chambers suggests that the authority of testimonial writing on AIDS "derives from the actual death of an actual author—an event on which the transformation of 'I am dying' into 'I is dead' hinges" (4).

8. This is, of course, a paraphrase of Susan Sontag's often-quoted formulation of one's

inherently dual citizenship "in the kingdom of the well and in the kingdom of the sick" (*Illness as Metaphor* 3).

9. The sheer bulk of research in autobiographical studies precludes a comprehensive reference. For representative perspectives of the two sides of the mentioned debate see Paul de Man's "Autobiography as De-facement" (1979), Michael Sprinkler's "Fictions of the Self" (1980), and Robert Elbaz's "Autobiography, Ideology and Genre Theory" (1988); compare with James Olney's *Metaphors of Self* (1972), Janet Varner Gunn's *Autobiography* (1982), and Paul John Eakin's "Self-Invention in Autobiography" (1989), *Touching the World* (1992), and his inspiring and innovative *How Our Lives Become Stories* (1999). In using the term *autobiography,* I draw on G. Thomas Couser's loose explanation that autobiography "by definition involves self-representation" ("Introduction" [2000] 305).

10. In a much-quoted statement, de Man asserted that, in autobiography, "whatever the writer *does* is in fact governed by the technical demands of self-portraiture and thus determined, in all its aspect, by the resources of his medium" ("Autobiography as De-facement" 920).

11. Tobin Siebers defines the weak sense of social constructionism as positing "that the dominant ideas, attitudes, and customs of a society influence the perception of bodies" ("Disability in Theory" 738). Prejudices of sex, gender, race, and ability are accounted for by human weaknesses of ignorance or misunderstanding rather than by the ideology of representation itself, as in the strong sense of social constructionism, where "the sign precedes the body in the hierarchy of representation" (739).

12. This claim has some affinities with Eakin's discussion of the embodied self in the first chapter of *How Our Lives Become Stories,* where he presents the new biological and psychological agreement on "the role of the body in the process of individuation" (17). Eakin has employed Oliver Sacks's and John M. Haull's narratives of disability to illustrate his claim that, even though our body image is "normally inaccessible to conscious examination and representation" (32), it functions as a baseline in our daily lives. For Eakin, these two narratives present a rare meeting ground for narrated and phenomenological experience; my own position is that all illness narratives grapple with the normally concealed body image as a result of their collapsed embodied identity and sense of self.

13. The terms *category, member,* and *nonfocal* are borrowed from Carolyn B. Mervis and Eleanor Rosch's research in cognitive psychology, in particular "Categorization of Natural Objects" (1981), which uses empirical findings to support the argument that the boundaries of categories are fuzzy rather than determinate or well defined.

14. G. Thomas Couser (*Recovering Bodies*) and Anne Hunsaker Hawkins (*Reconstructing Illness*) are the two major spokespersons for this claim. Their respective positions on the conventional narrative and cultural patterns used to ascribe meaning to illness are discussed in detail in chapter 1.

1 ILLNESS AS LIFE AFFAIR IN GILLIAN ROSE'S *LOVE'S WORK*

1. G. Thomas Couser and Ann Hunsaker Hawkins have contributed enormously to our understanding of the generic features of illness narratives, examining, respectively, the poetic devices and cultural myths pathographies usually employ.

2. This plot is defined by Arthur Frank in *The Wounded Storyteller* as "restitution narrative." Howard Brody notes that not only does the general public like these narratives, but "physicians especially like to tell them because [restitution] narratives have the happiest endings" (85).

3. Such thematic and formal features include numerous instances of intertextual "borrowing," such as citations of poems by Swinburne and Yeats; a full-fledged analysis of the Australian film *Picnic at Hanging Rock;* a direct quotation, as from a character's mouth, of a short Midrash story; and a quotation from Alexander Herzen's *My Past and Thought* that addresses the question of who is entitled to write his reminiscences. Many of these citations, furthermore, are there because they mattered to Rose's friends, thus emphasizing her concern with intersubjectivity and the connection between literature and love. Intersubjectivity is also evident in the two whole chapters that narrate the last phases of illness and the death of two of Rose's friends, which, in a way, mediates and amplifies her own thoughts on dying. Finally but not exhaustively, a remarkable literary allusion is introduced through an implicit analogy between Rose's formative experience of stealing a hymnal as a child and Rousseau's famous purloined ribbon.

4. Couser and Hawkins are agreed that the genre of illness narratives still awaits its masterpieces (Couser, *Recovering Bodies* 292; Hawkins 159). Couser adds, moreover, that little of the writing he surveyed in *Recovering Bodies* "may prove to have lasting value as literature in the traditional sense—books that require and reward rereading and close analysis" (292). To my mind, Rose's autobiography both requires and rewards such reading procedures, and, indeed, deserves to be appreciated as a masterpiece.

2 FIRST YOU HURT

1. See in particular Iris Marion Young, *Justice and the Politics of Difference* (1990), 139–41 (abbreviated in the text as *Justice*); Judith Butler's engagement with Irigaray's essay "Plato's Hysteria" (published in Irigaray's *Speculum of the Other Woman*) in *Bodies That Matter* (1993), 35–49; Elizabeth Grosz, *Volatile Bodies* (1994), 3–14 (abbreviated in the text as *VB*); Susan Bordo's "Introduction: Feminism, Western Culture, and the Body" in *Unbearable Weight* (1993); and Luce Irigaray's historical inquiry into Western metaphysics and science in "Is the Subject of Science Sexed?" (1989).

2. A good bibliography is provided in Kathy Davis's "Embody-ing Theory" (1997), 1–28 (abbreviated in this chapter as "Embody-ing"). Pertinent feminist analyses of Western science's neglect of the body as a product of the dualisms of Cartesian thought and the centrality of rationality in modernist science are provided by Susan Bordo in *The Flight to Objectivity* (1987); Evelyn Keller Fox in *Reflections on Gender and Science* (1985); and Moira Gatens in *Imaginary Bodies* (1996).

3. The various critical ramifications of this cultural transformation of the body are usefully sketched by Thomas J. Csordas in his "Introduction: The Body as Representation and Being-in-the-World" (1994).

4. AIDS activism, propelled forth by feminist and lesbian/gay involvement in liberatory identity politics, is the most recent example that springs to mind. On grassroots work done

by women with breast cancer at women's cancer resource centers, see Jackie Winnow's "Lesbians Evolving Health Care" (1991).

5. These emancipatory movements not only "assert[ed] the legitimacy of marginalized cultures and suppressed perspectives but also . . . expose[d] the biases of the official accounts [which now] had to be seen . . . as the products of historically situated individuals with very particular class, race, and gender interests" (Bordo, *Unbearable Weight* 219).

6. In chapter 2 of her *Justice and the Politics of Difference,* Young analyzes five aspects of cultural oppression: exploitation, marginalization, powerlessness, cultural imperialism, and violence (48–65).

7. Cultural imperialism as defined by Young "involves the universalization of a dominant group's experience and culture, and its establishment as the norm" (*Justice and the Politics of Difference* 59).

8. I am indebted to Toril Moi for this idea. See especially Moi's close reading of Butler's conception of materiality in *Gender Trouble* and *Bodies That Matter,* and her critique of the question of the materiality of the body raised by Butler as a problem produced by the poststructuralist picture of sex and gender (Moi 30–59, 73–77).

9. See Roseanne Lucia Quinn's "Mastectomy, Misogyny, and Media" (1995). Quinn observes "the dichotomization" practiced by academic feminists "of what women do, say, think, and write into opposing and mutually exclusive camps of 'theory' versus 'practice'" (268). She notes, further, the "similarly disturbing dichotomization . . . between the poststructuralists who tend to devalue experiential knowledge and those feminists who still talk about women as having real lives, with real bodies" (268). As David Morgan and Sue Scott have admonished in "Bodies in a Social Landscape" (1993), the new postmodernist theorizing of the body "has all too often been a cerebral, esoteric, and ultimately, disembodied activity" (18–19; qtd. in Davis, "Embody-ing," 14). See also Moi's critique of feminist poststructuralist theories on the body, which she finds "obscure, theoreticist, plagued by internal contradictions, mired in unnecessary philosophical and theoretical elaborations, and dependent on the 1960s sex/gender distinction for political effect" (58–59).

10. Here as elsewhere in this chapter, Toril Moi's exploration of Simone de Beauvoir's concept of the body as a situation in *The Second Sex* has been my constant inspiration. De Beauvoir's idea that the body *is* a situation (rather than that it is *in* a situation) is traced by Moi to Merleau-Ponty's project of showing that "in so far as the human body in concerned, one can draw no clear-cut line between that which belongs to the realm of nature and that which belongs to the realm of meaning." Moi further claims that, for both Merleau-Ponty and de Beauvoir, "the relationship between body and subjectivity is neither necessary nor arbitrary, but contingent" (114). See also Gatens's point that the relationship between the body and the psyche is contingent (*Imaginary Bodies* 13; ref. in Moi 82). While I embrace the definition of the relation between bodies and subjectivity as contingent, in my view the situation of the diseased body calls for adding the element of contiguity to this relation.

11. See Susie Orbach's *Hunger Strike* (1993) for the problematic consequences women's view of their bodies as commodities has for their body image. Kathryn Morgan, in "Women and the Knife" (1991), discusses women's conformity to traditional male-dominated ideologies of how women's bodies should look. Susan Brownmiller argues in *Femininity* (1985)

NOTES TO PAGES 41–47

that the impossible standards set by the system of beauty norms compel women's constant—and futile—engagement in the effort to attain a perfect body, thus ensuring their social subordination. Susan Bordo's study of cultural representations of women's bodies in film, advertising, and television in *Unbearable Weight* calls attention to the complex and durable strategies of social control that discipline and normalize the female body.

12. In *Body Image* (1999), Sarah Rogan provides sociological evidence of the overwhelming majority of British women who are dissatisfied with their bodies regardless of age and socioeconomic background.

13. Davis borrows this phrase from Dorothy Smith's *Texts, Facts and Femininity* (1990), in which femininity is viewed as a skilled activity.

14. Young does not pursue, however, her observation that "many women identify their breasts as themselves, living their embodied experience at some distance from the hard norms of the magazine gaze" (192). Rather, she attempts to minimize the significance of the alienated structure of the male gaze by juxtaposing it with "a construction, an imagining" of a woman's point of view of the breasted body as "blurry, mushy, indefinite, multiple, and without clear identity" (192–93). In spite of these gushing adjectives, her project of conceptualizing a woman-centered experience of breasts remains as abstract and detached from the concrete meanings of lived experience as the alienating male gaze she has condemned.

15. Sandra Steingraber relies on data provided by the National Cancer Institute and cited in *Harper's* "Index" (*Harper's* March 1990, 19). For a more recent confirmation of the scant progress in the cure rate of breast cancer see Alison Abbott's "On the Offensive" in *Nature* 4 April 2002. Abbott affirms that while up to 90 percent of childhood leukemias are now curable, mortality rates for "the big cancer killers—including breast, lung, prostate and colon cancers" have changed little since 1990 up to and including 2000 (470; see also figure on p. 473). The data currently available shows that more women died of breast cancer in 2000 than in 1990.

16. See Allen Jeffner and Iris Marion Young, eds., *The Thinking Muse* (1989).

17. See Weiss's valuable presentation of Merleau-Ponty's and Paul Schilder's work on the psychic development of body image and its enormous significance in lived experience, in "Body Image Intercourse: A Corporeal Dialogue between Merleau-Ponty and Schilder" (*Body Images* 7–38). In chapters 3 and 4 of *Volatile Bodies,* Elizabeth Grosz examines and critiques Schilder's and Merleau-Ponty's phenomenological studies of the body image and subjectivity from a feminist-psychoanalytic perspective (62–111).

18. From a different perspective, G. Thomas Couser refers to such stereotyped stories as manifesting "the tyranny of the comic plot." "Because disability is considered 'downbeat' or 'depressing,'" he says, "its representation may be allowed [by editors and publishers] only on the condition that the narrative take the form of a story of 'triumph'" ("Introduction" [2000] 308).

19. To my mind, this is the proper answer to Howard Brody's surprise at how different testimonies of sick people are in terms of the treatment preferences that they express (Brody, *Stories of Sickness,* 124–25). Being a sick person is no more monolithic a category than being a healthy person.

20. Marshall borrows this phrase from Alison Caddick's "Feminism and the Body" (1986) and "Feminist and Postmodern" (1992).

21. In his *Phenomenology of Perception* (1954), Merleau-Ponty argues that "[i]t is impossible to superimpose on man a lower layer of behaviour which one chooses to call 'natural', followed by a manufactured cultural or spiritual world" (189; qtd. in Moi 70). This claim complements from a phenomenological perspective the major contribution of poststructuralist philosophy in exposing the illusion of the metaphysic of a unified, self-making subjectivity that, as Young has said, "posits the subject as an autonomous origin or an underlying substance to which attributes of gender, nationality, family role, intellectual disposition, and so on might attach" (*Justice and the Politics of Difference* 45).

3 CONFESSING AIDS

1. These discourses, as Thomas Yingling has noted, are "variously comprised of the viral, the personal, the communal, the national, and the global" (292). For a discussion of cultural discourses as inseparable from and controlling the ways that AIDS has been framed by science, see Paula A. Treichler's "AIDS, Gender, and Biomedical Discourse."

2. Susan Sontag observed in *AIDS and Its Metaphors* that "to get AIDS is precisely to be revealed, in the majority of cases, as a member of a certain 'risk group,' a community of pariahs. The illness flushes out an identity that might have remained hidden from neighbors, jobmates, family, friends" (24–25).

3. My guess is that both the confessional mode and the politically charged connection Brodkey constructs between homosexuality and illness are accountable for this critical oversight. As one of the readers for this book, Ross Chambers, commented, "the confessional manner, with its insistence on shame, was unlikely to meet with much readerly complicity at a time when activists and others were desperately committed to combatting the stigmatization of AIDS and AIDS people." The only academic publication I have encountered so far that relates, albeit cursorily, to *This Wild Darkness*—Neil Small's "Death of the Authors"—altogether ignores the substantial parts of the text that discuss sexuality. On the other side of things, the book reviewer R. Baird Shuman insists on the autobiography's "virulent homophobia that [Brodkey] never acknowledges but that shows itself in numerous small ways throughout the book" (3). Beside these publications and a few brief descriptions of content, such as Eva Hoffman's in the *New York Times Book Review,* which appeared shortly after Brodkey's death, and apart from Robert Dessaix's rather derisive review in his collection (*and so forth*), there has been no interest, academic or otherwise, in Brodkey's *This Wild Darkness*.

4. Thomas G. Couser, *Recovering Bodies* 42. See also my discussion in chapter 1 of the conventions of illness narratives.

5. Brodkey's "monumental ego" and "legendary self-absorption" are also noted in R. Baird Shuman's review of *This Wild Darkness*.

6. Personal accounts of the embodied experience of dying have been discussed from ethical and social, mythological, and generic and narratological perspectives, respectively, by Arthur Frank *in The Wounded Storyteller,* Anne Hunsaker Hawkins in *Reconstructing Illness,* and G. Thomas Couser in *Recovering Bodies*.

7. For a discussion of Brodkey's distinctive narrative style see "Harold (Roy) Brodkey" in *Contemporary Novelists,* 6th ed., and "Harold (Roy) Brodkey 1930–1996" in *Contemporary Authors Online.*

8. For a comprehensive summary of relatively recent views on the connections between biology and culture see David B. Morris, *Illness and Culture in the Postmodern Age.*

9. Mary Gordon, "The Strangest Place to Be," review of *Tiger's Eye: A Memoir,* by Inga Clendinnen, 10.

10. Since Foucault's perspective of the evolution of discourses identifies the confessional mode as the foundational discourse of self-examination practices, a precursor of "the most highly valued techniques of producing truth" (*Introduction* 59), it follows that, for Foucault, any autobiographical discourse shares this status. As I have mentioned, however, it is important to note that while the "strong constructionists" among literary and cultural critics picked up this version of the confessing self, Foucault himself, as he was growing ill, drew back from this radical position. In volume 3 of *The History of Sexuality* (*The Care of the Self*), composed in the last years of his life, he tried to create a version of resistance to the hegemony of social power relations by developing a personal theory of taking care of the self, modeled on classical Greek and Roman sources.

11. Gilmore argues, further, that "the legacy of the confession for autobiography can be introduced as a history of valuing and devaluing, of determining and misrecognizing the profoundly political dimension of all discourses of identity" (*Autobiographics,* 108).

12. More specifically, as Frances Bartkowski has argued in "Epistemic Drift in Foucault," Foucault's talk about the possibility of resistance remains abstract and abstracted from actual experience: "The confession of which Foucault speaks at length is an attempt to give voice to the resistance: yet what we (readers/confessors) hear are not the voices of women, children, homosexuals, perverts, but the voice of power as it institutionalizes, rationalizes, domesticates, and suppresses those very discourses by which it shores itself up" (49; qtd. in Bernstein 31). To my mind, this critique applies as well to Foucault's famous dictum that "where there is power, there is resistance" (Foucault, *Introduction,* 95). It also holds true for Foucault's ideas on the possibility of resistance in *Power/Knowledge.* Thus, as Terence Turner has argued, once we accept Foucault's general view that "discourses and acts of resistance are themselves *really* forms of the 'power' which they imagine themselves to be resisting," we come to discredit "any possibility of a genuinely political or emancipatory criticism, let alone political action, of 'resistance'" ("Bodies and Anti-Bodies," 39). It was only much later in his life, significantly, when he himself became ill, that Foucault dealt directly with the experience, rather than the abstraction, of personal resistance.

13. Thus, Brodkey's sense of his irresistibility—which sustains his tacit belief that he in fact seduced his stepfather and subsequent abusers—is not unique but rather shared by many other abused children who were sexually assaulted within the family. In *The Secret Trauma,* Diana E. H. Russell observes that therapists who treat victims of incest often meet with projection of incestuous feelings by adult family members onto the abused children. Russell explains that accusations by fathers and other male relatives of a girl's (here: a boy's) seductive behavior serve as a rationalization for acting on sexual feelings. She emphasizes that "[e]ven the widespread use of the word *seduce* in this context is an offensive misnomer.

It assumes a mutuality—if not initially, then once the child has submitted. But the notion that a father *could* seduce, rather than violate, his daughter [or son] is itself a myth. And the notion that some daughters [or sons] seduce their fathers is a double myth" (392). As Brodkey's text shows all too well, sexually abused sons are prone to internalize this "double myth" of seduction as well as daughters, blaming their own behavior or tracing the abuse to a personal flaw inherent in themselves.

14. See John C. Gonsiorek, Walter H. Bera, and Donald LeTourneau, *Male Sexual Abuse*, 17.

15. *Pneumocystis carinii* pneumonia is the most common life-threatening opportunistic infection in AIDS patients. Eve K. Nichols, in *Mobilizing against AIDS*, says that the first signs of this disorder are "moderate to severe difficulty in breathing, dry cough, and fever" (45). Whereas the prospect of living with AIDS is much better today than when Brodkey wrote his AIDS memoir, in 1996 the accepted medical wisdom was that "[a]bout a fifth of AIDS patients who respond[ed] to therapy for *Pneumocystis carinii* relaps[ed], and those who [did] not eventually succumb[ed] to another infection" (Nichols 46).

16. The experience of the alien presence of the body in disease is discussed by Drew Leder in terms of "dys-appearance" in *The Absent Body* (82–99).

4 FLESH-TINTED FRAMES

1. The indexical elements of the medium of photography seem self-evident. After all, photography's mode of production consists of printing real objects on special subtonics through a combination of light and chemical action (photography literally means "writing with light"). Evidently, this definition applies only to traditional analogous photography, and not to digital photography or the translation of the photograph into digital information by use of a scanner. For a still-relevant discussion of the challenges posed to photography's capacity for reliable transcription by the application of computer technology, see Fred Ritchin's "Photojournalism in the Age of Computers."

2. See Allan Secula's "Dismantling Modernism" and Victor Burgin's "Looking at Photographs" and "Photography, Phantasy, Function." For a more focused discussion of the way the classical Renaissance system of single-point monocular perspective was built into camera optics from its infancy, thus neutralizing the position of visual mastery conferred upon the spectator, see Jean-Louis Baudry's "Ideological Effects of the Basic Cinematographic Apparatus" and Joel Snyder's "Picturing Vision." I was referred to these texts by Abigail Solomon-Godeau in "Who Is Speaking Thus? Some Questions about Documentary Photography."

3. Even critics who acknowledge the superior evidentiary value of photographs over paintings identify the reality effect of photography as suspect. Thus, Timothy Dow Adams, in *Light Writing and Life Writing*, writes that "[a]pparently no amount of appealing to logic about the obvious distortions of photographs can quite sway viewers from the popular idea that there is something especially authentic or accurate about photographic likeness" (4). Throughout his book, while Adams marks the historically enduring ambivalence of the status of photography since its invention, he maintains the view that the photographic tension between the staged and the real stems from our irrational faith in the magic of

photographic transcription. This chapter takes a different approach and theorizes the reality effect of illness photographs in rhetorical and narrative terms rather than in terms of "faith" or "magic."

4. *Cultural Sniping* will be henceforth abbreviated in the text as *CS*. A wealth of other informative materials by and about Spence exist in unpublished form as unnumbered papers at the Jo Spence Memorial Archive in London. I am indebted to the curator, Terry Dennett, for providing me with most of the unpublished documents and images relevant to Spence's work with illness and self-representation.

5. The Cancer Project comprises of a group of images Spence prepared for a retrospective exhibition showing the progress of her illness and her reactions to it over a period of nine years.

6. The citation is from the chapter "Identity and Cultural Production: Or Deciding to Become the Subject of Our Own Histories Rather Than the Object of Somebody Else's" (*CS* 129–36), which is a reprint of an article Spence published in the U.S. photography journal *Views* in 1990.

7. An overview of Spence's 1970s socialist interests is found in her article "Photography, Ideology and Education," which she coauthored with Terry Dennett. The essay focuses on photography as an educational tool and presents analytical and practical strategies through which to expose "the contradictions inherent in the present liberal teaching of history, which is a total rationalisation for past and present violence, the appropriation of the wealth, resources, land and labour of others, and various forms of cultural imperialism" (54).

8. See Raymond Williams's historical account of the development of the term *realism* in *Keywords*.

9. See note 6.

10. The caption was first added to Spence's Cancer Project exhibit in Nottingham, 1982.

11. "Questioning Documentary Practice? The Sign as a Site of Struggle," reprinted as a chapter in *Cultural Sniping* (97–108), was originally given as a keynote address at the first National Conference of Photography, organized by the Arts Council of Great Britain, in Salford, on 3 April 1987.

12. Terry Dennett was Spence's close friend and professional collaborator for most of her adult life. The citation is taken from a private correspondence with Dennett through electronic mail (12 September 2000).

13. Terry Dennett, e-mail to the author, 12 September 2000. Dennett's militant vocabulary here fits Jessica Evans's Foucauldian interpretation of Spence's 1985–86 project "The Picture of Health?", which evolved from these pictures (and from The Cancer Project as a whole). That project, says Evans, "makes visible in Foucauldian fashion those 'micro-capillary' forms of power which in touching the body are made corporeal" (240). Yet in 1984, when the photographs were created, Spence was ostensibly interested in creating Brechtian dramatic distancing and defamiliarizing effects in accord with the Russian Formalist tradition and its later development by Augusto Boal. For a discussion of the critical tradition that influenced Spence's documentary practice, see Terry Dennett and Jo Spence's "Making Strange Making New."

14. The essay from which the phrase is cited, "The Picture of Health? Part 3," is the third

in a three-part series of articles about cancer that originally appeared in the feminist magazine *Spare Rib* in 1986 and was reprinted in *CS.*

15. This quotation and the long quotation that immediately follows appear in chapter 25 of *CS,* which is a reprint of an interview conducted in 1991 between Jan Zita Grover and Jo Spence and originally titled "The Artist and Illness."

16. In "An Afterward and a Warning from Terry Dennett," Dennett observed that after her diagnosis, Spence had been warned by physicians that she would have only a year to live if she did not go through mastectomy and radiotherapy. "These predictions," says Dennett, "grew less credible as the patients of these specialists (the recipients of the very best radiation, chemicals and surgery that money could buy) began to die." Although her cancer recurred eighteen months after the lumpectomy, Spence managed to stabilize it through alternative treatment and enjoyed eight productive and relatively healthy years before she became ill again in 1990, with leukemia.

17. Here I refer to the initiation of Spence's interest in the method of phototheater in her 1982 show The History Lesson (also called Remodelling Photo History), which she coproduced with Terry Dennett. The show featured Spence, sometimes in the nude, in a series of seven previsualized, overtly political images meant to be used as an educational wedge against sexist, racist, and class assumptions. See *CS* (76–86) for a reprint of Spence's article "Remodelling Photo-History," which was first published in 1983, and in which she proposes to use these photographs in teaching photographic and art courses and workshops. The photographs were shown as part of a larger exhibition called Ten Contemporary British Photographers (Massachusetts Institute of Technology, February 1982). For a bright poststructuralist analysis of one of these photographs, *Colonization,* see Siona Wilson's article "White Metonymy."

18. This quoted passage was first published in Spence's interview with Jan Zita Grover, "The Artist and Illness." See note 15 and the works cited section for specific publication information.

19. The full quotation Jo Stanley seems to refer to is as follows: "I who had spent three years (and more) immersed in the study of ideology and visual representation now suddenly needed a new type of knowledge; [that] which has come to be called 'really useful social knowledge.' I realized with horror that my body was not made of photographic paper, nor was it an image, or an idea . . . it was made of blood, bones and tissue. Some of them now appear to be cancerous. And I didn't even know where my liver was" (Captions to *Mammogram,* Jo Spence/Terry Dennett/unknown radiographer, n.d., Jo Spence Memorial Archive, London.)

20. The citations refer, respectively, to the interview with Jan Zita Grover and to Spence's essay, "Identity and Cultural Production." See notes 15 and 6 and the works cited section for details of original publication.

21. The quotation is from Terry Dennett's "Notes on 'The Final Project,'" the unfinished essay that concludes *Cultural Sniping.* It was written in August 1994 and compiled by Terry Dennett in Jo Spence's Memorial Archive.

22. See note 21.

23. In one of his e-mail messages, Dennett discussed *Metamorphosis* as "unique in that

this is the only one of its type we could do, but it is not so in general terms if you consider [that] it really comes from the genre of 'last Will and Testament' which is also a pre and post death collaboration. In this case, between the deceased and their legal advisor via a Will" (E-mail to the author, 15 August 2000). Accordingly, the treatment, basic feature (i.e., a picture of Spence's head), and themes of the photograph were prescribed by Spence. Dennett's role was restricted to the actual selection of the basic image from the photographs included in Spence's photo-diary.

24. The quotation is taken from the caption beside Spence's photograph as it appears in *Cultural Sniping* (226).

25. Barthes' photographic paradox is discussed in detail in chapter 5.

26. The quotation is taken from Spence's "Identity and Cultural Production." See note 6 and the works cited section for publication details.

5 HANNAH WILKE: PERFORMING GRIEF

1. See my discussion of Harold Brodkey's account of AIDS in chapter 3, which employs Butler's category of "the constitutive outside" also as an explanatory concept of the experience of unmediated pain.

2. Myers's sister Joanne died from breast cancer, and his wife, Stephanie, is "a ten year survivor of the disease and one of the women [photographed] in the book" (Preface).

3. One of Saunders's major claims in *The Nude* is that since "[a]s a genre the female nude . . . has no purpose beyond the more or less erotic depiction of nakedness for male consumption" (23), the very oblivion of the woman to the spectator plays a significant role inasmuch as it leaves the viewer "free to gaze at her body and to fantasize about it unchallenged" (24).

4. The sleeping pose, as Saunders has observed, is a common device in representations of the nude female since it conveniently allows the viewer to enjoy the erotic spectacle of the woman's body while displacing the blame of voyeurism onto the provocative negligence of the woman herself. Here, however, the unresolved tension between picture and text disrupts the neutralizing effect of the photograph and calls for a deconstructive reading of the exclusive and productive visual strategies by which illness has been normalized.

5. In chapter 8, "Documentary Photography," of his book *The Photograph,* Graham Clarke provides a useful survey of the tradition and myths of documentary photography since its inception in Jacob Riis's pioneering photographs of the 1890s. Clarke focuses on the documentary photographer's political and aesthetic plotting of his or her subject, which ironically results in producing iconic objects of universal symbolic meaning (145–66). In "Who Is Speaking Thus?" Abigail Solomon-Godeau specifically posits the question of "whether the documentary act does not involve a double act of subjugation: first in the social world that has produced its victims; and second, in the regime of the image produced within and for the same system that engenders the conditions it then re-presents" (176). Even though, in the following essay, "Reconstructing Documentary," Solomon-Godeau examines the work of Connie Hatch as an example of contemporary documentary photography's success in self-consciously engaging in the dynamic operations of the act of looking, this kind of articulation of the a priori hierarchical relation between the photog-

rapher and her object is not a sufficient condition to cancel out the given hierarchy between the viewer and the viewed.

6. See Eleanor Rosch's "Principles of Categorization," in which she defines *prototype* as "the clearest cases of category membership defined operationally by people's judgments of goodness of membership in the category" (36).

7. The terms *focal* and *non-focal* were coined by Brent Berlin and Paul Kay in their 1969 investigation of focal and nonfocal colors in *Basic Color Terms*. Carolyn B. Mervis and Eleanor Rosch extend the usage of the nonfocal to their concept of the gradients of representativeness out of which all categories are composed. Specifically, they argue that the nonfocal nature of category membership can account for the fuzzy boundaries of categories that various empirical experiments demonstrated. See "Categorization of Natural Objects."

8. Abigail Solomon-Godeau, in "Who Is Speaking Thus?" (180), and Graham Clarke throughout his discussion of the history of photography in *The Photograph* are two relatively recent examples of critics who continue to use the terms *denotation* and *connotation* to explain photographic significance, although their historicist and deconstructive approaches resist the status of photography as, phenomenologically, a pure image.

9. John Tagg points at the psychological motivation behind Barthes' insistence on the photograph's evidential force. Thus, he says, Barthes' "demand for realism is a demand, if not to have [his mother] back, then to know she was here" (1). From a different perspective, Christian Metz observes that *Camera Lucida* bears witness to photography's "deeply rooted kinship with death" by "its position of annunciation . . . since the work was written just after (and because of) the death of the mother, and just before the death of the writer" (157).

CONCLUSION

1. Merleau-Ponty's argument in *Phenomenology of Perception* is that "[o]ur lives are not always lived in objectified bodies, for our bodies are not originally objects to us. They are instead the ground of perceptual processes that *end* in objectification" (7). While I have doubts concerning the developmental and linear definition of "original," "pre-objective" bodily experience, my reading of illness narratives has shown that embodied experience and knowledge are thrust upon the sick individual in ways that not only are "non-objectified" but often generate profound changes in previously held concepts about the body and the embodied self.

2. See Bruno Latour's *Science in Action,* referred to by Ineke Klinge in "Female Bodies and Brittle Bones." Klinge makes the parallel observation that "biomedical knowledge cannot directly 'mirror' natural reality. On the contrary, the production of scientific knowledge is a human enterprise and in accordance with operative norms and values—in short, with social-cultural conditions. Consequently, scientific knowledge has to be considered as historical and local" (59).

3. The exception that proves the general rule is Christine Battersby's work on a model of embodied identity and bodily boundaries in terms that draw from new topological the-

ories, such as catastrophe theory and chaos theory. See "Her Body/Her Boundaries" in *The Phenomenal Woman.*

4. Patrick Bateson and Paul Martin's *Design for a Life* is a comprehensive and highly enjoyable presentation of the interactive dynamics among a diversity of environmental and biological conditions that depend on but can in turn modify the mechanisms in the brain responsible for learning and other forms of behavior. The methodology and working paradigms of bioepistemology are discussed in Nancy Easterlin's "Making Knowledge."

WORKS CITED

Abbott, Alison. "On the Offensive." *Nature* 4 April 2002: 470–74.

Adams, Timothy Dow. *Light Writing and Life Writing: Photography in Autobiography.* Chapel Hill: University of North Carolina Press, 2000.

Altman, Denis. *AIDS in the Mind of America.* 1986. Garden City, NY: Anchor Books, 1987.

Barthes, Roland. *Camera Lucida: Reflections on Photography.* Trans. Richard Howard. New York: Hill and Wang, 1986.

———. "The Photographic Message." *Image/Music/Text.* Trans. Stephen Heath. New York: Hill and Wang, 1977. 15–31.

———. "Rhetoric of the Image." *Classic Essays in Photography.* Ed. Alan Trachtenberg. New Haven: Island Books, 1980. 269–85.

Bartkowski, Frances. "Epistemic Drift in Foucault." *Feminism and Foucault.* Eds. Irene Diamond and Lee Quinby. Boston: Northeastern University, 1988. In Bernstein 31.

Bartky, Sandra. *Femininity and Domination: Studies in the Phenomenology of Oppression.* New York: Routledge, 1990.

Bateson, Patrick, and Paul Martin. *Design for a Life: How Behaviour Develops.* London: Jonathan Cape, 1999.

Battersby, Christine. "Her Body/Her Boundaries." *The Phenomenal Woman: Feminist Metaphysics and the Patterns of Identity.* New York: Routledge, 1998. 38–60.

Baudry, Jean-Louis. "Ideological Effects of the Basic Cinematographic Apparatus." 1970. Rpt. in *Movies and Methods* Vol. 2. Ed. Bill Nichols. Berkeley: University of California Press, 1985. 531–42.

Berlin, Brent, and Paul Kay. *Basic Color Terms: Their Universality and Evolution.* Berkeley: University of California Press, 1969.

Bernstein, Susan David. *Confessional Subjects: Revelations of Gender and Power in Victorian Literature and Culture.* Chapel Hill: North Carolina University Press, 1997.

Bordo, Susan. *The Flight to Objectivity: Essays on Cartesianism and Culture.* Albany: SUNY Press, 1987.

———. *Unbearable Weight: Feminism, Western Culture, and the Body.* Berkeley: University of California Press, 1993.

Brodkey, Harold. *This Wild Darkness: The Story of My Death.* New York: Metropolitan Books, 1996.

Brody, Howard. *Stories of Sickness.* 2nd ed. Oxford: Oxford University Press, 2003.

Brownmiller, Susan. *Femininity.* New York: Fawcett Columbine, 1985.

Burgin, Victor. "Looking at Photographs." *Thinking Photography.* Ed. Victor Burgin. London: Macmillan, 1982. 142–53.

———. "Photography, Phantasy, Function." *Thinking Photography.* Ed. Victor Burgin. London: Macmillan, 1982. 177–216.

Butler, Judith. *Bodies That Matter: On the Discursive Limits of "Sex".* New York: Routledge, 1993.

Caddick, Alison. "Feminism and the Body." *Arena* 74 (1986): 60–90.

———. "Feminist and Postmodern." *Arena* 99/100 (1992): 112–28.

Chambers, Ross. *Facing It: AIDS Diaries and the Death of the Author.* Ann Arbor: University of Michigan Press, 1998.

Clarke, Graham. *The Photograph.* Oxford History of Art. Oxford: Oxford University Press, 1997.

Couser, G. Thomas. "Introduction to the Empire of the 'Normal': A Forum on Disability and Self-Representation." *American Quarterly* 52.2 (2000): 305–10.

———. *Recovering Bodies: Illness, Disability, and Life Writing.* Madison: University of Wisconsin Press, 1998.

Coward, Ross, and Jo Spence. "Body Talk? A Dialogue between Ross Coward and Jo Spence." *Photography/Politics: Two.* Eds. Patricia Holland, Jo Spence, and Simon Watney. London: Comedia/Photography Workshop, 1986. 24–39.

Csordas, Thomas J. "Introduction: The Body as Representation and Being-in-the-World." *Embodiment and Experience: The Existential Ground of Culture and Self.* Ed. Thomas J. Csordas. Cambridge: Cambridge University Press, 1994. 1–26.

Dansky, Steven F. *Now Dare Everything: Tales of HIV-Related Psychotherapy.* New York: Harington Park Press, 1994.

Davis, Kathy. "Embody-ing Theory: Beyond Modernist and Postmodernist Readings of the Body." *Embodied Practices: Feminist Perspectives on the Body.* Ed. Kathy Davis. London: Sage Publications, 1997. 1–28.

———. "'My Body Is My Art': Cosmetic Surgery as Feminist Utopia?" 1997. Rpt. in Price and Shildrick, *Feminist Theory* 444–65.

———. *Reshaping the Female Body: The Dilemma of Cosmetic Surgery.* London: Routledge, 1995.

WORKS CITED

Davis, Lennard J. *Bending over Backwards: Disability, Dismodernism, and Other Difficult Positions.* New York: New York University Press, 2002.

de Man, Paul. "Autobiography as De-facement." *Modern Language Notes* 94 (1979): 919–30.

———. "The Purloined Ribbon." 1977. Rpt. as "Excuses (Confessions)." *Allegories of Reading.* New Haven: Yale University Press, 1979. 278–301.

Dennett, Terry. "An Afterward and a Warning from Terry Dennett." 1995. N. pag. Jo Spence Memorial Archive, London.

———. "Notes on 'The Final Project: A Photo Fantasy and Phototherapeutic Exploration of Life and Death,' 1991–92." *Cultural Sniping,* by Jo Spence. London: Routledge, 1995. 222–23.

———. "PhotoTherapy—PhotoTheatre: Jo Spence's Innovative Autobiographic Uses of Photography." 1997. N. pag. Jo Spence Memorial Archive, London.

———, and Jo Spence. "Making Strange Making New." 1991. N. pag. Jo Spence Memorial Archive, London.

Dessaix, Robert. "The Story of Harold Brodkey's Death." *(and so forth).* Sydney: Pan Macmillan, 1998. 93–97.

Eakin, Paul John. *How Our Lives Become Stories: Making Selves.* Ithaca: Cornell University Press, 1999.

———. "Self-Invention in Autobiography: The Moment of Language." *Fictions in Autobiography: Studies in the Art of Self Invention.* Princeton: Princeton University Press, 1989. 181–278.

———. *Touching the World: Reference in Autobiography.* Princeton: Princeton University Press, 1992.

Easterlin, Nancy. "Making Knowledge: Bioepistemology and the Foundations of Literary Theory." *Mosaic* 32.1 (1999): 131–40.

Elbaz, Robert. "Autobiography, Ideology and Genre Theory." *The Changing Nature of the Self: A Critical Study of the Autobiographic Discourse.* London: Cromm Helm, 1988. 1–16.

Evans, Jessica. "An Affront to Taste? The Disturbances of Jo Spence." *The Camerawork Essays* 237–61.

———, ed. *The Camerawork Essays: Context and Meaning in Photography.* London: Rivers Oram Press, 1997.

Foster, Dennis A. *Confession and Complicity in Narrative.* Cambridge: Cambridge University Press, 1987.

Foucault, Michel. *The History of Sexuality: An Introduction. Volume 1.* Trans. Robert Hurley. 1978. Rpt. New York: Vintage Books, 1990.

———. *The History of Sexuality: The Care of the Self. Volume 3.* Trans. Robert Hurley. New York: Random House, 1986.

Fox, Evelyn Keller. *Reflections on Gender and Science.* New Haven: Yale University Press, 1985.

Frank, Arthur W. *The Wounded Storyteller: Body, Illness, and Ethics.* Chicago: University of Chicago Press, 1995.

Gatens, Moira. *Imaginary Bodies: Ethics, Power, and Corporeality.* New York: Routledge, 1996.

Gilmore, Leigh. *Autobiographics: A Feminist Theory of Women's Self-Representation.* Ithaca: Cornell University Press, 1994.

———. "The Mark of Autobiography: Postmodernism, Autobiography, and Genre." *Autobiography and Postmodernism.* Eds. Kathleen Ashley, Leigh Gilmore, and Gerald Peters. Amherst: University of Massachusetts Press, 1994. 3–18.

Goddard, Donald. "Life Drawings." *Intra-Venus.* 3rd ed. New York: Ronald Feldman Fine Arts, 1995. 16.

Gonsiorek, John C., Walter H. Bera, and Donald LeTourneau. *Male Sexual Abuse: A Trilogy of Intervention Strategies.* London: Sage Publications, 1994.

Gordon, Mary. "The Strangest Place to Be." *New York Times Book Review* 26 August 2001: 10.

Grosz, Elizabeth. "Bodies-Cities." *Space, Time, and Perversion: Essays on the Politics of Bodies.* New York: Routledge, 1995. 103–10.

———. "Psychoanalysis and the Body." 1992. Rpt. in Price and Shildrick, *Feminist Theory* 267–71.

———. *Volatile Bodies: Toward a Corporeal Feminism.* Bloomington: Indiana University Press, 1994.

Gunn, Janet Varner. *Autobiography: Toward a Poetics of Experience.* Philadelphia: University of Pennsylvania Press, 1982.

Haraway, Donna. "The Biopolitics of Postmodern Bodies: Determinations of Self in Immune System Discourse." Price and Shildrick 203–14.

"Harold (Roy) Brodkey." *Contemporary Novelists,* 6th ed. Ed. Susan Windisch Brown. Detroit: St. James Press, 1996. 149–50.

"Harold (Roy) Brodkey, 1930–1996." *Contemporary Authors Online.* Gale Group: 2002. http://galenet.com/servlet/GLD/hits . . . o&1=d&locID=columbiau&NA= Harold+Brodkey.

Hawkins, Anne Hunsaker. *Reconstructing Illness: Studies in Pathography.* West Lafayette: Purdue University Press, 1993.

Hess, Elizabeth. "Self- and Selfless Portraits." *Village Voice* 26 September 1989: 93. Qtd. in Jones 4.

Hirsch, Marianne. *Family Frames: Photography, Narrative, and Postmemory.* Cambridge, MA: Harvard University Press, 1997.

Hoffman, Eva. Rev. of *This Wild Darkness: The Story of My Death,* by Harold Brodkey. *New York Times Book Review* 27 October 1996: 7–9.

Howells, William Dean. "Autobiography: A New Form of Literature." *Harper's Monthly* 119 (Oct. 1909): 798. Qtd in Couser, "Introduction" 305.

Irigaray, Luce. "Is the Subject of Science Sexed?" *Feminism and Science.* Ed. Nancy Tuana. Bloomington: Indiana University Press, 1989. 58–68.

Isaak, Jo Anna. "In Praise of Primary Narcissism: The Last Laughs of Jo Spence and Hannah Wilke." *Interfaces: Women, Autobiography, Image, Performance.* Eds. Sidonie Smith and Julia Watson. Ann Arbor: University of Michigan Press, 2003. 49–68.

Jeffner, Allen, and Iris Marion Young, eds. *The Thinking Muse: Feminism and Modern French Philosophy.* Bloomington: Indiana University Press, 1989.

Jones, Amelia. "*Intra-Venus* and Hannah Wilke's Feminist Narcissism." *Intra-Venus.* 3rd ed. New York: Ronald Feldman Fine Arts, 1995. 4–13.

Klinge, Ineke. "Female Bodies and Brittle Bones: Medical Interventions in Osteoporosis." *Embodied Practices: Feminist Perspectives on the Body.* Ed Kathy Davis. London: Sage Publications, 1997. 59–72.

Krauss, Rosalind. "A Note on Photography and the Simulacral." *The Critical Image: Essays on Contemporary Photography.* Ed. Carol Squiers. Seattle: Bay Press, 1990. 15–27.

Latour, Bruno. *Science in Action: How to Follow Scientists and Engineers through Society.* Cambridge, MA: Harvard University Press, 1987. Ref. in Klinge 59.

Leder, Drew. *The Absent Body.* Chicago: University of Chicago Press, 1990.

———. "Introduction." *The Body in Medical Thought and Practice.* Ed. Drew Leder. Dordrect: Kluwer Academic Publishers, 1992. 1–12.

Lejeune, Philippe. *On Autobiography.* Edited with a foreword by Paul John Eakin and translated by Katherine Leary. Minneapolis: University of Minnesota Press, 1989.

Lippard, Lucy. "The Pains and Pleasure of Rebirth: European and American Women's Body Art." *From the Center: Feminist Essays on Women's Body Art.* New York: E. P. Dutton, 1976. Qtd. in Jones 5.

Lorde, Audre. *The Cancer Journals.* San Francisco: Aunt Lute Books, 1980.

Mairs, Nancy. *Waist-High in the World: A Life among the Nondisabled.* Boston: Beacon, 1996.

Marshall, Helen. "Our Bodies, Ourselves: Why We Should Add Old Fashioned Empirical Phenomenology to New Theories of the Body." 1996. Rpt. in Price and Shildrick, *Feminist Theory* 64–75.

Mayer, Musa. *Examining Myself: One Woman's Story of Breast Cancer Treatment and Recovery.* Boston and London: Faber, 1993.

Merleau-Ponty, Maurice. *Phenomenology of Perception.* 1954. Trans. Colin Smith. London: Routledge, 1962.

Mervis, Carolyn B., and Eleanor Rosch. "Categorization of Natural Objects." *Annual Review of Psychology* 32 (1981): 89–115.

Metz, Christian. "Photography and Fetish." *The Critical Image.* Ed. Carol Squiers. Seattle: Bay Press: 1990. 155–64.

Middlebrook, Christina. *Seeing the Crab: A Memoir of Dying before I Do.* 1996. New York: Anchor Books and Doubleday, 1998.

Mitchell, W. J. T. *Picture Theory: Essays on Verbal and Visual Representation.* Chicago: Chicago University Press, 1994.

Moi, Toril. *What Is a Woman?* Oxford: Oxford University Press, 1999.

Morgan, David, and Sue Scott. "Bodies in a Social Landscape." *Body Matters*. Eds. Sue Scott and David Morgan. London: Falmer Press, 1993. 1–21.

Morgan, Kathryn. "Women and the Knife: Cosmetic Surgery and the Colonization of Women's Bodies." *Hypatia* 6 (1991): 25–53.

Morris, David B. *Illness and Culture in the Postmodern Age*. Berkeley: University of California Press, 1998.

Murphy, Robert F. *The Body Silent: The Different World of the Disabled*. New York: W. W. Norton, 1990.

Myers, Art. *Winged Victory: Altered Images Transcending Breast Cancer*. San Diego: Photographic Gallery of Fine Art Books, 1996. N. pag.

Nagy, Gregory. "The Crisis of Performance." *The Ends of Rhetoric: History, Theory, Practice*. Eds. John Bender and David E. Wellbery. Stanford: Stanford University Press, 1990. 43–59.

Nichols, Eve K. *Mobilizing against AIDS: The Unfinished Story of a Virus*. Cambridge, MA: Harvard University Press, 1986.

Olney, James. "Autobiography and the Cultural Moment: A Thematic, Historical, and Bibliographical Introduction." *Autobiography: Essays Theoretical and Critical*. Ed. James Olney. Princeton: Princeton University Press, 1980. 3–27.

———. *Metaphors of Self: The Meaning of Autobiography*. Princeton: Princeton University Press, 1972.

Orbach, Susie. *Hunger Strike: The Anorectic's Struggle as a Metaphor for Our Age*. London: Penguin, 1993.

Parker, Lisa S. "Beauty and Breast Implantation: How Candidate Selection Affects Autonomy and Informed Consent." *Feminist Ethics and Social Policy*. Eds. Patrice Diquinzio and Iris Marion Young. Bloomington: Indiana University Press, 1997. 252–73.

Pessoa, Fernando. "Self-Analysis." *Self-Analysis and Thirty Other Poems*. Trans. George Monteiro. Lisbon: Calouste Gulbenkian Foundation, 1988.

Phelan, James. *Narrative as Rhetoric: Technique, Audiences, Ethics, Ideology*. Columbus: Ohio State University Press, 1996.

Price, Janet, and Margrit Shildrick. "Breaking the Boundaries of the Broken Body." 1996. Rpt. in Price and Shildrick, *Feminist Theory* 432–44.

———, eds. *Feminist Theory and the Body: A Reader*. New York: Routledge, 1999.

Quinn, Roseanne Lucia. "Mastectomy, Misogyny, and Media: Toward an Inclusive Politics and Poetics of Breast Cancer." *Violence, Silence, and Anger: Women's Writing as Transgression*. Ed. Deirdre Lashgari. Charlottesville: University Press of Virginia, 1995. 267–81.

Ricoeur, Paul. *The Symbolism of Evil*. Trans. Ned Lukacher. Baltimore: Johns Hopkins, 1982.

Ritchin, Fred. "Photojournalism in the Age of Computers." *The Critical Image: Essays on Contemporary Photography*. Ed. Carol Squiers. Seattle: Bay Press, 1990. 28–37.

WORKS CITED

Rogan, Sarah. *Body Image: Understanding Body Dissatisfaction in Men, Women and Children.* London: Routledge, 1999.

Rorty, Richard. *Contingency, Irony, and Solidarity.* Cambridge: Cambridge University Press, 1989.

Rosch, Eleanor. "Principles of Categorization." *Cognition and Categorization.* Eds. Eleanor Rosch and Barbara B. Lloyd. Hillsdale, NJ: Lawrence Erlbaum, 1978. 27–48.

Rose, Gillian. *Love's Work: A Reckoning with Life.* London: Chatto and Windus, 1995. Rpt. New York: Schocken Books, 1996.

Rosen, Roee. "Less and More than Two." *Beauty Is a Promise of Happiness.* Jerusalem: Israel Museum, 1996. 1–5.

Rosenblum, Barbara, and Sandra Butler. *Cancer in Two Voices.* 1991. Duluth, MN: Spinsters Ink, 1996.

Roth, Jay S. *All about AIDS.* Chur, Switzerland: Harwood Academic Publishers, 1989.

Russell, Diana E. H. *The Secret Trauma: Incest in the Lives of Girls and Women.* New York: Basic Books, 1986.

Said, Edward W. "The Problem of Textuality: Two Exemplary Positions." *Critical Inquiry* 4.4 (1978): 673–714.

Saunders, Gill. *The Nude: A New Perspective.* New York: Harper and Row, 1989.

Scarry, Elaine. *The Body in Pain.* 1985. Rpt. New York: Oxford University Press, 1987.

Secula, Allan. "Dismantling Modernism: Reinventing Documentary." 1978. Rpt. in *Photography against the Grain.* Halifax: Press of the Nova Scotia College of Art and Design, 1985. 53–76.

———. "On the Invention of Photographic Meaning." 1975. Rpt. in *Photography in Print: Writings from 1816 to the Present.* Ed. Vicki Goldberg. New York: Simon and Schuster, 1981. 452–73.

Sedgwick, Eve Kosofsky. "White Glasses." *Tendencies.* London: Routledge, 1994. 252–66.

Shavid, Ariela. *Beauty Is a Promise of Happiness.* Jerusalem: Israel Museum, 1996.

Shuman, R. Baird. Rev. of *This Wild Darkness: The Story of My Death,* by Harold Brodkey. *Magill Book Reviews* 1 August 1997: 3.

Siebers, Tobin. "Disability in Theory: From Social Constructionism to the New Realism of the Body." *American Literary History* 13.4 (2001): 737–54.

Small, Neil. "Death of the Authors." *Mortality* 3.3 (1998): 215–29.

Smith, Bruce R. "Premodern Sexualities." *PMLA* 115.3 (2000): 318–29.

Smith, Dorothy. *Texts, Facts and Femininity: Exploring the Relations of Ruling.* London: Routledge, 1990.

Smith, Sidonie, and Julia Watson. "Introduction: Mapping Women's Self-Representation at Visual/Textual Interfaces." *Interfaces: Women, Autobiography, Image, Performance.* Eds. Sidonie Smith and Julia Watson. Ann Arbor: University Of Michigan Press, 2003. 1–46.

Snyder, Joel. "Picturing Vision." *The Language of Images.* Ed. W. J. T. Mitchell. Chicago: University of Chicago Press, 1980. 219–58.

Solomon-Godeau, Abigail. "Who Is Speaking Thus? Some Questions about Documentary Photography." 1986. Rpt. in *Photography at the Dock: Essays on Photographic History, Institutions, and Practices*. Minneapolis: University of Minnesota Press, 1997. 169–83.

Sontag, Susan. *Illness as Metaphor; and AIDS and Its Metaphors*. 1978, 1989. Rpt. New York: Anchor Books and Doubleday, 1990.

Spence, Jo. *Cultural Sniping: The Art of Transgression*. Eds. Jo Stanley and David Hevey. London and New York: Routledge, 1995.

———. "Identity and Cultural Production." *Views* (Summer 1990). Rpt. as "Identity and Cultural Production: Or Deciding to Become the Subject of Our Own Histories Rather Than the Object of Somebody Else's" in Spence, *Cultural Sniping* 129–36.

———. "The Picture of Health? Part 3. " *Spare Rib* 165 (April 1986). Rpt. in Spence, *Cultural Sniping* 113–23.

———. *Putting Myself in the Picture: A Political, Personal, and Photographic Autobiography*. Seattle: Real Comet Press, 1988.

———. "Questioning Documentary Practice? The Sign as a Site of Struggle." Keynote address at the National Conference of Photography. Salford, Great Britain. 3 April 1987. Rpt. in Spence, *Cultural Sniping* 97–108.

Spence, Jo, and Terry Dennett. "Metamorphosis." 1995. N. pag. Jo Spence Memorial Archive, London.

———. "Photography, Ideology and Education." *Screen Education* 21 (1977): 42–69.

———. "Remodelling Photo-History: An Afterword on a Recent Exhibition." *Screen* 23.1 (1983). Rpt. in Spence, *Cultural Sniping* 76–86.

Spence, Jo, and Jan Grover Zita. "The Artist and Illness: Cultural Burn-out/Holistic Health! (Interview with Jan Grover Zita)." *Artpaper* (1991). Rpt. in Spence, *Cultural Sniping*, 212–17.

Sprinkler, Michael. "Fictions of the Self: The End of Autobiography." *Autobiography: Essays Theoretical and Critical*. Ed. James Olney. Princeton: Princeton University Press, 1980. 321–42.

Steingraber, Sandra. "Lifestyles Don't Kill. Carcinogens in Air, Food, and Water Do: Imagining Political Responses to Cancer." *Cancer as a Women's Issue: Scratching the Surface*. Ed. Midge Stocker. Chicago: Third Side Press, 1991. 91–102.

Sutton, John. *Philosophy and Memory Traces: Descartes to Connectionism*. Cambridge: Cambridge University Press, 1998.

Tagg, John. *The Burden of Representation: Essays on Photographies and Histories*. Minneapolis: University of Minnesota Press, 1988.

Turner, Terence. "Bodies and Anti-Bodies: Flesh and Fetish in Contemporary Social Theory." *Embodiment and Experience: The Existential Ground of Culture and Self*. Ed. Thomas J. Csordas. 1994. Cambridge: Cambridge University Press, 2000. 27–47.

Treichler, Paula A. "AIDS, Gender, and Biomedical Discourse." *AIDS: The Burdens of*

History. Eds. Elisabeth Fee and Daniel M. Fox. Berkeley: University of California Press, 1988. 190–266.

———. "Escaping the Sentence: Diagnosis and Discourse in 'The Yellow Wallpaper.'" *Feminist Issues in Literary Scholarship.* Ed. Shari Benstock. Bloomington: Indiana University Press, 1987. 62–78.

Weiss, Gail. *Body Images: Embodiment as Intercorporeality.* New York: Routledge, 1999.

Wendell, Susan. "Feminism, Disability, and the Transcendence of the Body." 1996. Rpt. in Price and Shildrick, *Feminist Theory* 324–33.

Wilber, Treya Killam, and Ken Wilber. *Grace and Grit: Spirituality and Healing in the Life and Death of Treya Killam Wilber.* Boston: Shambhala, 1993.

Wilke, Hannah. *Intra-Venus Series, Photographs. Portraits with Donald Goddard,* 1991–1992. *Intra-Venus.* 3rd ed. New York: Ronald Feldman Fine Arts, 1995.

Williams, Raymond. *Keywords.* Glasgow: Fontana, 1976. Rpt. New York: Oxford University Press, 1983.

Wilson, Siona. "White Metonymy: A Discussion around Jo Spence and Terry Dennett's Colonization." *Third Text* 37 (1996–97): 3–15.

Winnow, Jackie. "Lesbians Evolving Health Care: Our Lives Depend on It." *Cancer as a Women's Issue: Scratching the Surface.* Ed. Midge Stocker. Chicago: Third Side Press, 1991. 23–37.

Wittman, Juliet. *Breast Cancer Journal: A Century of Petals.* Golden, CO: Fulcrum Publishing, 1993.

Yingling, Thomas. "AIDS in America: Postmodern Governance, Identity, and Experience." *Inside Out: Lesbian Theories, Gay Theories.* Ed. Diana Fuss. New York: Routledge, 1991. 291–310.

Young, Iris Marion. "Breasted Experience: The Look and the Feeling." *Throwing Like a Girl and Other Essays in Feminist Philosophy and Social Theory.* Bloomington: Indiana University Press, 1990. 189–209.

———. *Justice and the Politics of Difference.* Princeton: Princeton University Press, 1990.

INDEX

Page numbers in italics refer to illustrations.

Sontag, Susan, 85, 165n8, 170n2

Spence, Jo, 19, 99–101, 116–18, 139–40, 149, 151, 155, 158; *Alternative Health Treatment Using Traditional Chinese Medicine,* 110, *111;* The Cancer Project photographs, 101–16; *The Consultant's Ward Round,* 101, *102,* 103, 106; *Cultural Sniping,* 100; The Final Project, 118–24, 126–27; The History Lesson (Remodelling Photo History), 174n17; *Infantilization* series, 108–10, *109; Marked Up for Amputation,* 104–7, *107,* 109, 139; *Metamorphosis,* 119, *120,* 121–22, 124, 126–27; "The Picture of Health?",* 112, 173n13; *Untitled* (1992), 124, *125; Write or Be Written Off, 114,* 115–16

Stanley, Jo, 174n19

structuralist criticism, 19

Sutton, John, 160–61

Tagg, John, 149, 153–54, 176n9

temporal shifts, 19, 97–98, 140, 153, 155

truth telling. *See* confession

Turner, Terence, 93, 171n12

van Pelt, Robert Jan, 35–36

Weiss, Gail, 60–61, 64, 160

Wendell, Susan, 44–47, 67

Wilber, Treya Killam, 11, 17, 46, 50, 67–68

Wilke, Hannah, 99–100, 129–40, 149, 151, 155; *Intra-Venus,* 19–20, 129–30; *Intra-Venus Series No. 1,* 131–33, *132; Intra-Venus Series No. 3, 136,* 137; *Intra-Venus Series No. 4, 134,* 135; *Intra-Venus Series No. 9, 133,* 134; *Intra-Venus Series No. 10,* 137, *137; Intra-Venus Series No. 12,* 135, *135; Brushstrokes,* 135; *Super-T-Art,* 130, *131*

Wittman, Juliet, 68

Yingling, Thomas, 85

Yordy, Charles, 82

Young, Iris Marion, 40, 41–42, 48, 168nn6–7